Praise for
Lose the Gluten, Lose your Gut.
Ditch the Grain, Save your Brain.

'Lose the Gluten, Lose your Gut, Ditch the Grain, Save your Brain,' is an informative piece written by Drs. Stephanie and Tom Chaney that is well-founded in the science of understanding the dangers of gluten in our diets. This book aims to answer questions like, "why is our population so unhealthy?" And, "why can't we lose weight?" Their book does just that and will astound you in the process.

My first reaction; why doesn't everyone know this? Because they should. I praise the Chaney's for taking the initiative to write this book, to tell their stories and to be proactive about what this substance of gluten is doing to the American population. They describe how gluten and grain intake have contributed to diseases like diabetes, thyroid and digestive dysfunctions.

Unlike many books I've read that were written by doctors, this book makes sense. They teach you how dangerous gluten is and how our everyday grains are synonymous with the substance. This is a topic that needs to be learned, discussed, thought and known by every family. Simply, Drs. Tom and Stephanie Chaney have written a practical guide to health, eating and the restoration of a long list of conditions.

~ **Dr. Richard Schmitt**
  CEO, CE4You
  Past President of the Maryland Chiropractic Association

"Lose the Gluten" is a tremendous resource for healthcare providers and the general public alike. In this comprehensive book, Drs. Stephanie and Thomas Chaney have done a remarkable job of clearly explaining how gluten can create a wide variety of health problems. Their book provides great information on not just all the food that contains gluten, but also provides extremely practical information on HOW to change your diet so that you can maximize your health through appropriate nutrition. Their evidence-informed approach yields a highly reputable yet easy to read guide on becoming a healthier human being. The Chaney's certainly identified a need and created a solution. I will positively recommend this to my friends, family and patients and know that it will enhance their lives. Thank you Dr. Stephanie and Thomas for creating such an amazing book!"

~ **Dr. Jay S. Greenstein**, DC, CCSP, CGF1-L1, CKTP, FMS
  CEO, Sport and Spine Companies

Over the past several decades, "whole wheat" and "fat-free" have become synonymous with "health food". As a natural health care practitioner, it is often an overwhelming task to re-program the thinking of my patients and encourage the lifestyle changes necessary for them to achieve true transformation. Thankfully, Drs. Chaney have provided an excellent roadmap to teach patients not only WHY they must change their diet, but also HOW. Over the last few years I have been an observer of the fantastic results Dr. Steph is getting in her practice and know that her program is based on solid science and that her commitment to her patients is second to none. This book, in my opinion, will become a valuable resource to any practitioner who wishes to guide his or her patients toward achieving greater health and wellbeing.

~ **Kay B. O'Hara, D.C., M.Ac.**
   Eastern Chiropractic
   Harmony Classical Acupuncture

Doctors Tom and Steph have really delivered the goods with their work in this book. Not only do they provide thorough research to show proof positive what gluten does to the body, they give you practical solutions, and even recipes, to make the transition to 'gluten-free' much easier. This book is a must-read for all healthcare providers so they can disseminate a holistic, natural solution to society's growing obesity epidemic.

~ **Dr. Bobbee Palmer, DC**
   Co-Founder - Chiropractic Business Academy
   www.chirobizacademy.com

In this day and age, many people are actively seeking resources that enable them to take better care of their bodies. This book is a definite must have if you are one of those people; not only for personal use, but also to keep in your lending library for the benefit of others. It is the small changes in our daily routine that often have the largest effect in our quality of life and possible longevity.

~ **Dr. Robert Berry**
   Chiropractic BioPhysics Advanced Certified & Instructor
   CEO of Berry Translations Equipment Company
   Private Practice- Montour Falls, New York

Drs. Stephanie and Tom Chaney are highly experienced Doctors of Chiropractic. They have put their years of practice, research and experience as well as passion to help improve people's health into this book.

This book will reveal truths about healthy living and how to change not only how you look on the outside but change the actual biochemistry and function of your body on the inside.

A for sure must read. You will be more aware, healthier and happier you have this information.

~ Dr. Stephanie Higashi, D.C.
President and Founder of Mar Vista Health Center and Health Atlast

---

Drs Tom and Stephanie Chaney are true pioneers in the field of Gluten. Not only are they well versed about the research and practice-based health risks and dangers associated with gluten, they LIVE the way they encourage their patients to live, leading people by example and demonstrating how gluten-free eating is a pleasure. The recipes and their food plans are easy to follow and delicious!

~ Dr. Renee Sacharny

This book contains vital data for anyone interested in having a healthy body. Every person on the planet makes several daily food choices and without this information they are at risk! I have independently researched many of the topics covered in this book and have adopted a lifestyle consistent with what Drs. Tom and Steph discuss herein—resulting in a resurgence in my energy, health and happiness. As a doctor interested in your health and as a friend interested in your well-being I urge you to read this book as a first step towards improving conditions in your health and your life!

~ Eric R. Huntington, D.C.
Doctor of Chiropractic
Healthcare Innovator and Consultant

I have read countless books on diet and gluten is now finally pinpointed as a recognized culprit for all kinds of physiological dysfunction and overall lowered health status. Drs. Chaney's give us a contemporary and well-rounded account of gluten and its health impact. A must read for anyone attempting to achieve total health and wellness in today's world!

~ **Paul Oakley, D.C., MSc**
  www.shotguntohealth.com

Patient Testimonials

All patient testimonies are real and the names have been abbreviated for privacy. No payment was made in exchange for these testimonials. This is just a sample of the thousands of testimonials that Drs. Chaney have received during years of practice.

I am in control of what I eat instead of food cravings controlling me.

~ Lisa C.

I was surprised that I wasn't hungry at all…I've lost inches everywhere and a substantial amount of weight.

~ Sandy S.

I no longer have days where I feel as if I am 'dragging'…Stomach aches are a thing of the past.

~ Misty M.

My blood levels are in the normal range with half of the medication.

~ Matthew P.

My A1C has gone from 9.4 to 6.2 and I'm feeling better than I have in years.

~ Karen B.

I lost 8 lbs. in the first 4 days.

~ Dianne G.

I love the weight loss-feeling great!

~ Luise F.

My blood sugar is below 100, I am off of 6 out of 8 prescribed medications, I have lost 16 pounds in 2 months.

~ Tony S.

I've seen an improvement in my weight, high blood pressure and my sugar levels.
~ Cora M.

My goal was to avoid complications later in life due to diabetes. I think I've achieved that. I've been able to eliminate 3 medications and reduce another. I have been to too many docs in the past only to receive more meds and bad news!

~ Jonathan H.

I wish that I had heard about Drs. Chaney 10 years ago. I would not have had to spend so many years gaining weight, being tired and feeling depressed.

~ Ollie G.

If someone had told me 3 months ago that I could give up gluten, grains, dairy and sugar all in a week and feel this great…I would have called them crazy!

~ Mary P.

Dr. Chaney helped me understand more about me and my health in these past few weeks, than other doctors have in years.

~ Herb W.

You've shown me the pathway to great health and what it takes to make a complete life change for me and my family's overall health.

~ Mallory B.

Within 3 weeks of the program I was off blood pressure meds!

~ Rajeev C.

My constant heart burn is gone, no more Zantac 4 times a day! After 20 years of pills and discomfort I finally feel as though there is light at the end of the tunnel.

~ Carole O.

Seeking out the professionals at Living Health is the best decision I have made in my adult life. Awesome!!

~ John R.

This treatment(program) turned my life around. I was in bad shape and struggling to function (with Hashimoto's) but now I have energy and know what foods to eat to stay that way.

~ Donna M.

He (Dr. Tom) lectured us on the remote causes of Diabetes and said that they will first tackle the remote causes, correct them and reverse the Diabetes. I am confirming that they did all of these and more.

~ Lyn U.

Lose the

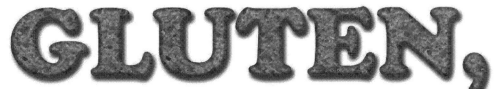

Lose your

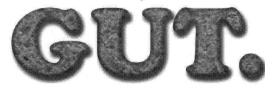

Ditch the

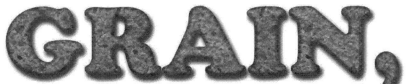

Save your

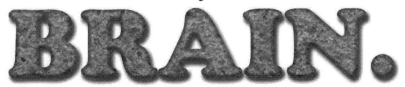

DISCOVER HOW GLUTEN AND "HEALTHY" WHOLE GRAINS
CONTRIBUTE TO OBESITY, TYPE 2 DIABETES,
ALZHEIMER'S DISEASE, AND OTHER DEADLY DISEASES..

**AND WHAT YOU MUST DO TO PREVENT
AND REVERSE THEM.**

Stephanie J. Chaney, DC & Thomas A. Chaney, DC

Lose The Gluten, Lose Your Gut. Ditch The Grain, Save Your Brain.

DISCOVER HOW GLUTEN AND "HEALTHY" WHOLE GRAINS CONTRIBUTE TO OBESITY, TYPE 2 DIABETES, ALZHEIMER'S DISEASE, AND OTHER DEADLY DISEASES..

AND WHAT YOU MUST DO TO PREVENT AND REVERSE THEM.

Stephanie J. Chaney, D.C.
Thomas A. Chaney, D.C.

Disclaimer: This information is intended as a reference volume only, not as a medical manual. The information given here is designed to help you make informed decisions about your health. The Author makes no representations or warranties with respect to the accuracy or completeness of the contents of this work and specifically disclaims all warranties, including without limitation warranties of fitness for a particular purpose. No warranty may be created or extended by sales or promotional materials. The advice and strategies contained herein may not be suitable for every situation. This Author shall not be liable for damages arising herefrom. This information is not intended as a substitute for any treatment that may have been prescribed by your doctor. The fact that a Doctor, organization or website is referred to in this work as a citation or source of information does not mean that the Author endorses the information the organization, the Doctor or website may provide or recommendations it may make. If you suspect that you have a medical problem, we urge you to seek competent medical help.

Printed by Selby Marketing Associates, Rochester, NY

Library of Congress Cataloging-in-Publication Data
Drs. Stephanie and Thomas A. Chaney, D.C.
Lose The Gluten, Lose Your Gut. Ditch The Grain, Save Your Brain. Discover how gluten and "healthy" whole grains contribute to obesity, type 2 diabetes, alzheimer's disease, and other deadly diseases..And what you must do to prevent and reverse them by Drs. Stephanie and Thomas A. Chaney, D.C. – 1st ed.
Includes references and index.
ISBN: 978-0-9854157-0-9

Library of Congress Number: 2012945795

Table of Contents

Foreword

In our current health care system, we see healthcare costs rising higher and higher every day, though we rarely know the reason why. The lucky among us work hard to get good jobs with health benefits to combat this rise in healthcare costs. Those benefits may not be options to every family, though, and may not cover the care that we actually need. More often people find that they're paying for care and treatments that they don't require or even want. The pill-after-pill model of care, after all, is probably not what we have in mind when it comes to our health.

Unfortunately, that's exactly what these expensive insurance providers pay for and suggest, and it's what they'll continue to pay for in our healthcare protocol.

This means that the very model of care we don't want is exactly what we're getting. There are a couple of reasons for this – it's easy on the insurance companies, and it's in fashion in the medical industry. When we talk to our friends and family about health and the state of the health care system, we may find that they're facing similar problems – they suffer from a number of complaints, including pain, diabetes, decreased sex drive, headaches, hair falling out ... you name it, and they have it. They're going to their healthcare providers about the problems, and discussing the options with their insurance companies, but not getting any definitive answers. More importantly, they're not seeing any improvement.

What they do get are excuses for the lack of improvement. Every ailment has a range of possible 'explanations.' Headaches are from stress at work. Hair falling out is because of that new conditioner you're using. You're tired because you wake up too early. Sex drive... well you know, it's all about age. As doctors we hear them all, and we may even offer them as possibilities at times. Through every situation like this, though, we hear the symptoms screaming that something is wrong. Something in the person's body is not working as it should. It's like we all start life getting straight A's, and then as time goes on we start dropping down until we're getting C's. There must be a reason for this drop off. And there must be something we can do.

We make excuses or we tell ourselves that it's not that bad. We may see other family and friends getting F's, and think "at least I am not that bad." We're quite a ways from that A we were once so proud of, but at least we're not as bad as some of the other people we know. At some point we all hit a wall. We hit a place in life where we decide we're not satisfied, and we do want to feel better. When we get to this point, we take that stand and go to our doctor saying I want to feel better!

What happens then? We're led on a path of test after test, and given drug after drug to "fix" us. Eventually we go into surgery to repair what's wrong. As time goes by, we lose more body parts to these surgeries and add more drugs to the cocktail to replace the natural processes we've lost or to boost them up in one way or another. We become victims of the chemical side effects of those drugs, and dependent on outside help. We become dismantled in our health and risk the time bomb of too much medication. Suddenly we've arrived at the F we thought we could avoid with the great insurance and medical treatment we've been paying for.

Eventually, after you visit doctor after doctor, all of whom studied under the same model of care, you'll come to realize that none of it is going to get you anywhere. The standard healthcare process dismantles you and makes you dependent, instead of making you better. At some point, you may begin to wonder how you got there in the first place. More importantly, you'll wonder whether you can go back – reverse the effects of the medications, surgeries, and treatments. You might not think you can. You might think that your path was set for you, via genetics and lifestyle. You might be reading all the health books and magazines trying to figure out whether you missed something or whether there was a simpler answer that you missed.

You may do what so many other people have done – trust those in the medical industry to take care of you regardless of what it's doing to your body. You may trust the marketers of the nation's food products assuming that they put the best possible products out there. You may save money by buying the lower quality food products on sale rather than the more expensive organic options. We don't expect any of this to be harmful. We certainly don't expect these decisions to be at the base of many of our health problems.

What we need to realize is that if these health problems are so common they might be stemming from something we all do. Maybe something that we all trust is not actually "trustworthy." We can start with the healthcare industry; perhaps finding a quality doctor is harder than we anticipate, since so much of a healthcare provider's advice is dictated by crummy emergency insurance coverage. We can move from there to the nutrition of our country; perhaps finding healthy food means looking for more than advertising and 'professional' advice. The reality is that the medical community is headed in the wrong direction for healthcare, while our food manufacturers are giving us products that may actually aggravate our health problems. These are two very important – and interconnected – pieces of our health puzzle.

If you're experiencing health problems and looking for ways to heal, there may be some very simple choices before you. There is no magic bullet or secret potion for better health, but there is common sense and pure science, which suggest that the food you're eating may be the reason you're feeling awful. The food that is being sold to you, so cheaply and easily, actually has devastating effects on your wellbeing. It's not complex. It's very simple, and as obvious as day.

Drs. Tom and Steph Chaney look into these possibilities, along with their short- and long-term effects, and give us a straight and clear answers to the questions we're facing. The text that follows will blow your previous ideas of health away, and open your eyes to a world of new information. The authors offer a simple and healthy way to understand a number of health problems, and tell you how to treat those problems at their root cause. With their expert advice and guidance, you'll find that making the change from an unhealthy lifestyle to a health lifestyle can be both quick and easy.

Your doctor might not want you to read this book. After all, changing your lifestyle through something as easy as altering your eating habits will eliminate the need for all that medication in your cabinet. This book doesn't follow the instructions the doctor has received from the insurance companies. It does offer you the best way forward to greater health and quality of life. For that reason alone this book belongs in every American kitchen.

Yours in health,

Dr. Jonathan Spages D.C.
Author of *The Wellness Approach: The Secrets to Health our Doctor is Afraid to Tell You!*

Introduction

The Organization for Economic Cooperation and Development published a report in 2010 stating that in almost half of the developed countries one out of every two people is overweight or obese. This report also projected that in some countries 2 out of every 3 people will be obese within ten years. In the United States, the Centers for Disease Control (CDC) found that 68 percent of the adult population is overweight and 28 percent is obese.[1] America has the dubious honor of leading the world with the fattest population of children. It has become obvious that when it comes to being healthy and living a healthy lifestyle we are losing the war.

In our years of practice we have seen thousands of patients. One of the first questions we ask each new patient is, "What are your health goals?" The most common answer that comes out of almost every person's mouth is, "I want to lose weight!" But how can this possibly be? There are so many "solutions" out there. There is a weight loss company on every corner and entire sections in bookstores are dedicated to diet and weight loss. Our country spends vast amounts of money on "health" care and every magazine in the grocery store has a least one article discussing diet and exercise. Many of our patients have tried these "solutions" but have not seen results. Waistlines, and medication lists, continue to grow and they are seemingly diagnosed with a new condition or disease upon each visit to the doctor.

There is no missing the fact that the world is fat and unhealthy. We are living the "fast food" lifestyle, eating what we want, when we want it and unfortunately suffering the consequences. Not only are we overweight, but we are fast becoming one of the most chronically ill countries on the planet. Furthermore, as leaders to other nations, we are spreading our ill-health globally via the Standard American Diet (SAD). These chronic illnesses include type 2 diabetes, heart disease, autoimmune diseases, etc. These illnesses also happen to be the top killers of our population. So, what is at the heart of this deadly pattern? In our opinion, the answer to this question is GLUTEN.

Part One:
What is Gluten and What's the BIG Deal?

Our Story

In the ten years that we have been in practice helping patients improve their health, the areas of focus in the practice have evolved. Our passion has always been to help patients improve their health naturally, without pharmaceuticals or surgery if possible. Over the last five years, the development of functional medicine in our practice has evolved and expanded. Thus, we have helped patients overcome a variety of conditions. Prior to, and along with this practice evolution, has come much professional development, education and training. Each time we learn something with proven clinical relevance we apply it to our patient care, and also to ourselves. We learned about comprehensive testing that is typically not done in the conventional health care setting, and began screening our patients for, among many things, gluten reactivity and gluten-related disorders.

Dr. Tom on Dr. Steph's health

When we took note of how prevalent gluten reactivity and gluten-related disorders were with our patients, it became apparent that we should get ourselves tested as well. Although we had no intestinal issues (or so we thought), Dr. Steph had been diagnosed at the age of 9 with juvenile rheumatoid arthritis, an often debilitating and disfiguring autoimmune disease whereby the immune system begins to attack the joints as though knees, knuckles and elbows were enemy invaders.

It came on one night as an intense full-body attack of joints throughout her body. Her joints were so swollen and painful that she couldn't roll over to get out of bed. She had to be carried into the hospital. For years, she would suffer from attacks to seemingly random joints that would last for months.

Due to the fact that Dr. Steph is autoimmune, she is more likely to develop autoimmunity to other tissues, such as that of the thyroid, the pancreas and the brain, than someone who has not yet become autoimmune. Since wheat and gluten is a trigger for intestinal permeability, sometimes referred to as "Leaky Gut Syndrome," a condition which may ultimately trigger autoimmunity to commence or flare-up, we were very interested in pursuing a gluten-free lifestyle. By doing so, we hoped Dr. Steph would remain in remission for the rest of her life.

Since childhood, Dr. Steph has worked very hard to naturally stop her disease in its tracks. Dr. Steph has never been on medication for her rheumatism, even through some painful flare-ups. She has been in remission for almost 20 years after making key changes to her diet and lifestyle – one of them being the elimination of gluten. Working passionately to be naturally healthy is what motivated Dr. Steph to become a chiropractor – a true case of "patient, heal thyself" by becoming her own doctor!

Dr. Steph on Dr. Tom's health

As for Dr. Tom, the "healthy" one with no specific complaints, we were shocked that his testing came back "off the charts" positive for non-celiac gluten sensitivity/reactivity. We immediately cut gluten out of our diet. Due to my personal battle with rheumatism, which enstilled good eating habits, Dr. Tom's gluten-free diet was not a huge stretch for us. Dr. Tom's body was having an immune reaction each and every time he ingested gluten and he didn't even know it!

Since Dr. Tom didn't suffer from any of the intestinal symptoms that are common for those with Celiac disease, and because he went to the gym and exercised regularly, slept well and had good energy, he didn't expect to even notice a difference after eliminating gluten. Boy, was he wrong.

Immediately after removing gluten he began to observe the positive impact on his health. The biggest changes he noticed were an increase in energy and much less fatigue during the day. The knee pain that he had had for years completely disappeared. He didn't lose weight, but lost inches in the waist and went down 2 pants sizes. He also noticed improved mental focus and concentration. Was it possible that his gluten reaction caused him to attack his joints and brain tissue, leaving his gut relatively symptom-free? How scary is that thought?

Dr. Tom began to discuss gluten-related disorders with family members. His father has a history of heart disease, has had heart surgery and is on medications. He also complains of joint pain and inflammation. We sent him for testing and sure enough he also tested positive for non-celiac gluten sensitivity/reactivity. We put him on a program to eliminate gluten, decrease inflammation and repair his gut. He has completed the program and his doctor has taken him off all of his medications, he lost 40 pounds, has more energy and less joint pain. In our opinion, and based on what we've read in the research, his gluten-related disorder contributed to his heart disease and overall state of inflammation. This is not a far-fetched concept since heart disease and other diseases such as diabetes are now understood to be inflammatory disorders. This small change has made a big difference in his life and his health.

Many people are concerned about genetics and hereditary diseases. We became very aware that Dr. Tom was traveling the same path as his father. Had it not been for the specialized education and training we received and by keeping up with the latest research, we would not have made this change. Dr. Tom would have suffered the consequences, and probably would have blamed a potential future heart attack on genetics and heredity, especially given how healthy our diet was compared to that of most people.

We truly believe that linking common everyday symptoms such as brain fog, headaches, memory lapses and fatigue to lifestyle choices, specifically to eating gluten and other grains, is very important for people to know since these 'no biggie' symptoms can be signs of serious trouble down the road, such as autoimmune diseases, Alzheimer's, Parkinson's, osteoporosis, heart disease, strokes, and even cancer.

Now, if Dr. Tom unintentionally consumes gluten, he knows right away. He is more aware of, and sensitive to, gluten exposures. The reactions vary, but usually he experiences extreme fatigue, sometimes a headache, bloating, gas and usually joint pain. These symptoms alone are enough for him to want to stay gluten-free, but even more of a motivation for him to remain gluten-free is to prevent, and avoid, the potentially life threatening, long-term effects of gluten-related disorders to which none of us is immune. We want to prevent heart disease, neurological and brain degenerative disorders and all of the other chronic diseases that have been linked to gluten-related disorders. We want to live a long, high quality and active life and we feel that making this change has given us the best opportunity to do that.

And, we want this for each and every patient with whom we work.

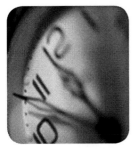

So how did we get here?

There has been an evolution in our society from that of a hunter-gatherer society to an agricultural lifestyle. The prehistoric hunter-gather diet, consumed by our ancestors, was higher in protein and fats from game meat and lower in carbohydrates, sugars and starches than that of the diet that we eat today.[2,3] This shift towards agricultural farming has led to a seemingly endless supply of refined foods and processed grains.[4] Humans have been eating grains, including wheat, for only an estimated 10,000 to 15,000 years. In the millions of years that humans have been evolving, that's really not that long. In fact, if you were to look at human existence along the timeline of a clock face, agriculture and grain-eating did not present until approximately 11:54 in a 12 hour cycle.

It wasn't until a couple hundred years ago that we began truly emphasizing single crops, hybridizing and intensely processing grains and isolating proteins from grains. It's only even more recently, within the last few decades, that we've also genetically modified many grains. As a result, the grains we consume today are not the grains we consumed a few thousand years ago or even a few generations ago. And, because of this, they are not the grains we as humans have developed the ability to digest and utilize for optimum nutrition! Some anthropology experts even go so far as to say that humans have never really had the ability to digest grains and should not have even started in the first place.[5]

It has been hypothesized by researchers that the opiate/morphine-like effects of grains is what caused us to 'settle down' from our previous hunter-gatherer ways, and is what allowed us to be less aggressive in general and more suited to civilization.[6] Yes, that's right, grains (wheat in particular) digest down to an opiate/morphine-containing chemical that affects our brains the same way that these commonly known drugs do. According to these researchers, this may partly explain the impetus to consume grains despite the disease- and discomfort-causing properties the grains had. These grains continue to have negative effects on human health and are not compatible with the human digestive system. We are simply not designed to digest these grains. We become nutrient and vitamin deficient when consuming grains because they are difficult to fully and efficiently digest and this inability to digest results in absorption issues within the gut. Potentially even worse, our immune systems can begin to react to grain proteins as though they were a foreign enemy, trying to attack and eliminate them as though they were a bacteria or virus. And this is part of the overall inflammatory problem—when the immune system reacts to these substances, it can end up harming our digestive systems, our nervous systems and our overall health.

Over the thousands of years that agricultural techniques have developed, and particularly in the last few hundred years, humans actively selected grains that reproduced and grew easily, and that produced higher yields of seeds and higher levels of protein. When we could no longer do this 'naturally,' scientists discovered ways to genetically alter the grains to produce even higher yields of proteins from the single grain "berry." From the farmer's point of view, this makes perfect sense—the farmer wants to get the most from his or her fields while minimizing the cost and potential problems. But, while the farmers were getting more efficient harvests, the grains were becoming more and more supersized with gluten and becoming even more "alien" to the human digestive system—and thus to the human immune system!

Moreover, these proteins are now being extracted from grains and processed into thousands of manufactured 'foods,' leading to an almost all-day-every-day exposure to gluten and other grain proteins, an assault that surely did not take place even 200 years ago, and one that causes immune reactions potentially on a 24/7 basis.

The patients coming in our office often have no idea about the amount of grain they consume in the average day. It is usually not until they write a diary of their diet that they see the servings of grains they are consuming each day, oftentimes upwards of 70-80% of their diet. There are a couple of reasons for this. One reason is because many patients do not know the difference between a grain and a vegetable. That is a problem. When asked what vegetables they like, the usual response typically includes corn. Unfortunately corn is not a vegetable, but a grain. Another reason for such high grain consumption is that many grains, and grain proteins, as stated earlier, are hidden from plain view and processed into foods that we wouldn't think would need to contain grains, and we consume them without us even knowing we are eating grains. These include salad dressings and other condiments – even chewing gum!

These patients have also been told—by the government (aka lobbyists), doctors, nutritionists and dieticians, the media, the internet, their personal trainer, or their neighbor, Joe - that they should eat more whole grains. The common recommendation patients have been told is to switch from the "white stuff" to "healthy," whole grains, because it is better for them. The problem is that it really doesn't make a huge difference because they are both grains that contain potentially disease-causing proteins. These are the same patients that start their day, each and every day, with oatmeal, cereal, toast or a bagel - all grains. They have been told that this is good for their heart and their cholesterol levels. Yet, there must still be a problem because they are still on cholesterol and blood pressure medication, and oftentimes, their health continues to decline.

Then we have the food pyramid, or more recently, the USDA "food plate." On the bottom of the "retired," but still commonly used food pyramid, the largest group is grains. The pyramid recommendation is 6-11 serving of grains per day. The newer recommendations, from "My Plate" still recommends that about ¼ of your diet should be grains. No wonder we are seeing the expanding waistlines! Especially, since most folks think that corn is a vegetable and are likely to insert corn in the veggie section, and eat rice, pasta or another grain in the grain section, and then not even count the bread roll sitting somewhere else on the table. If they kept the pyramid, they could have simply chopped off the lower section completely and we would have seen dramatic improvements in health versus what we're seeing now.

THEN:

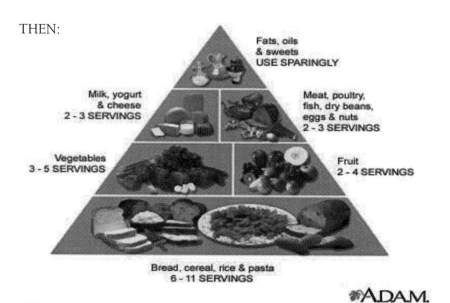

NOW:

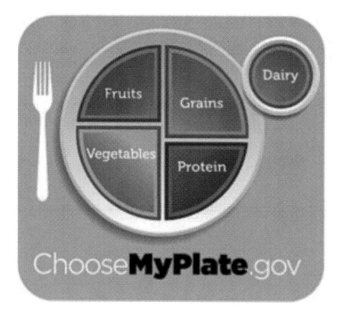

Common grain products:

Amaranth	Quinoa (not really a grain, but often eaten as one)
Corn	
Cornbread	Sorghum
Brown/White Rice	Pasta
Buckwheat	Flour Products/Cereals
Couscous (wheat-based)	Whole Wheat Products (white flour, etc.)
Bulgur	Rye
Millett	Spelt
Oatmeal	Barley
Rolled Oats	Teff

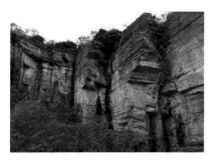

Food companies utilize many new grain-based ingredients in the manufacturing of almost all of our processed, pre-packaged foods. This results in an exposure to a variety of grain proteins that the human body has never experienced before. This leads to a constant, daily, bombardment of these grain proteins. This, combined with all the other stressors of modern life, has taken our immune systems to the edge of the proverbial cliff.

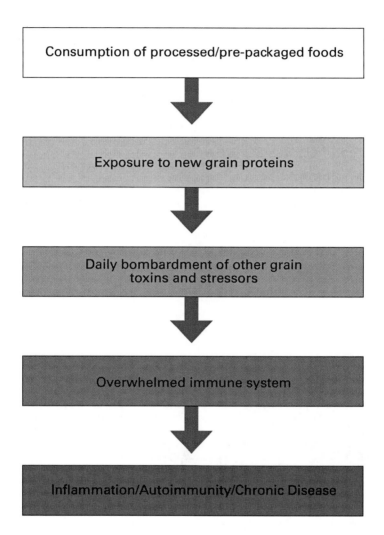

Many times people are not even aware that they are eating a grain. Most of us are being "educated" by either the marketing departments of the food distributors or by the pharmaceutical companies, which, it must be admitted, have some financial interests in people's health (or 'ill-health'). This makes it difficult to know the difference between what we should be eating to be healthy and prevent chronic disease and what companies are telling us to eat just to sell their products. Through intense lobbying efforts made by big agricultural companies and the food manufacturers, we are educated by a government that many of the population blindly trusts to tell us/educate us on what we can, and should, eat. A deadly mix if you ask us.

Let's list just a few examples of the epidemics other than obesity that are making their unfortunate mark.

- Autism rates are through the roof. In the 1980's, the estimate rate of autism was 1 in 2500. In the last few decades, that rate has increased to 1 in 150 children.[7,8] Of course, there are controversies concerning whether these statistics represent a "real" increase in the rate of autism, or if we are simply so much better at diagnosing autism. If it is your child, however, there is no controversy over how "real" the increase is![9]

- Type 2 diabetes, in combination with pre-diabetes is predicted to reach 50% of the population by 2020. The American Diabetes Association reports that currently, 8.3% of the entire population in the US has been diagnosed with diabetes—this includes children and adults. In 2010, nearly 2 million people were diagnosed. In persons older than 65, the percentage diagnosed with diabetes is nearly 27%! It should be mentioned here that diabetes is thought to be a process that starts with blood glucose (sugar) imbalances, insulin resistance, pre-diabetes and then progresses to full-blown diabetes. With this in mind, it is likely that the percentage of people with any of these pre-diabetic conditions is higher than the percentage of those diagnosed with diabetes. Think about what that might mean in your life!

- Heart disease has been the leading cause of death for over 80 years. This death rate has declined somewhat, mainly through an all-out "war" on heart disease. But, as the American Heart Association recently said: "...the Burden of Disease Remains High."[10] Interestingly, the American Diabetes Association states that 2 out of every 3 diabetics will die of a cardiac event (heart attack or stroke). Perhaps type 2 diabetes and heart disease, both inflammatory diseases, are one in the same...

- Cancer has likely touched everyone, either directly or indirectly, and is likely to continue doing so. According to the CDC, the leading cause of cancer deaths are lung, prostate, colon and liver cancers for men, and lung, breast and colon cancer for women.[11]
- Autoimmune diseases are also on the rise.[12] The reason for this increase is not fully understood by researchers but some of the contributing factors include genetics, environment and nutritional factors. The research shows that gluten-related disorder is a systemic autoimmune disease with diverse manifestations.[13] This increase in autoimmunity may also be correlated with Vitamin D deficiencies that seem to be related to the recommendations to limit sun exposure to limit skin cancer.[14] Autoimmune diseases such as Type 1 diabetes, is also related to and affected by nutrition, particularly nutrition in early childhood.[15,16] Other autoimmune diseases such as rheumatoid arthritis,[17,18] skin disorders, neurological disorders and digestive disorders can significantly improve on a gluten- and grain-free diet.[19,20,21] It has been estimated that autoimmune disease is the third leading cause of morbidity and mortality in the industrialized world.[22]

What you will learn by reading this book is that the diseases listed above are all, in some way, negatively impacted by, worsened by, or in many instances, caused by the inflammation triggered by **gluten exposure and reactivity.**.

It sometimes seems as if there is no end in sight with nearly everyone from birth on is suffering from one condition or another. But, you should know that all of these disorders are linked in some way with what we put in our mouths, every meal of everyday – and gluten-containing grains and other grains are at the center of it all.

It could be argued that the sum total of deaths resulting from heart disease, diabetes and autoimmunity might be caused by, or expedited by, continuous exposure to wheat and gluten in our modern day diets. Could it be that wheat- and gluten-reactivity, since it is the common denominator in all of these top-ranked diseases, is actually the number one cause of morbidity and mortality in the industrialized world, expressing itself in such a myriad of ways that we've been overlooking it the entire time?

What is gluten?

Gluten is a family of proteins—the name comes from the fact that this protein, found mainly in wheat, acts like "glue." It is the gluten in wheat that makes baked goods so gooey-gooey good and glues all of the ingredients together when baking. It is also the glue-like gluten that makes flour and water turn into a great cement for paper maché projects. It's this glue-like gluten that helps thicken sauces and gravies, and even helps give shampoo that goopey hold.

Wheat is the grain that happens to contain the highest amount of gluten. It contains even more gluten today than it did a few hundred years ago because it has been bred to yield larger quantities and more protein. Gluten can be found not only in wheat but also in rye, barley, spelt and some "ancient" grains.

Whole wheat itself, as well as gluten, causes inflammation of the intestinal lining and is implicated in the development of Increased Intestinal Permeability, also commonly known as Leaky Gut Syndrome.[23,24,25] Most people, however, are not reacting simply to wheat itself, but to one or more of the breakdown products (smaller proteins and peptides) that result from poor digestion of wheat. This is where the trouble starts. We will discuss more about this later.

Why all the hype over gluten?

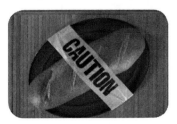

Have you noticed that the term "gluten-free" is showing up on food labels everywhere? Even chewing gum labels will advertise if the product is gluten-free. On a recent trip to Brazil for a conference, we noticed that everything from sugar packets to soda was labeled as gluten-free or not. We learned that one of the leading researchers of Parkinson's is a Brazilian medical doctor who has linked this devastating disease with gluten-reactivity.

So what's the big deal suddenly? Is this just marketing hype?

Most people, when they hear about gluten-related disorders, think that gluten-reactivity is something only those with Celiac disease have. Celiac disease is also known as "gluten-sensitive enteropathy." Enteropathy simply means disease of the gut. How does this disease develop? Celiac disease is an autoimmune disorder triggered by the ingestion of gluten and a resulting immune reaction to gluten in genetically predisposed people. The human leukocyte antigen (HLA) is associated with Celiac disease, specifically serotypes DQ2 and DQ8.[26,27] (An antigen is any substance that can cause an immune reaction) It is estimated that 40-50% of the population is a DQ2/DQ8 gene carrier (and therefore has a potential to develop Celiac disease).

Once wheat and/or gluten is ingested, it is poorly digested and this starts a cascade of inflammatory reactions in the intestinal lining. One of the 'positive' test markers a person must have in order to be diagnosed with Celiac disease is a significant antibody response to one of the gluten proteins or peptides.

Antibodies are the soldiers of the immune system. Antibodies are encoded to identify specific invading proteins or peptides. Once identified, the antibody neutralizes the invading protein or peptide so the body can safely dispose of it. In the case of the celiac or other gluten-reactive individual, antibodies are calibrated to identify specific gluten proteins or peptides. Some of these proteins digested down from wheat are similar to protein structures found in body tissues (such as the lining of the intestines)—and these antibodies may not simply 'attack' these wheat/gluten-derived proteins, but ultimately may also be triggered to destroy the lining of the intestines.

As a result of this antibody response and the damage to the intestines, many people, particularly those with Celiac disease, are unable to get the proper nutrients from their diet. The only treatment for Celiac disease is to permanently and completely avoid gluten. When people with Celiac disease adhere to the gluten-free diet, they can recover, or go into 'remission.'

Symptoms of Celiac disease include abdominal pain or discomfort, constipation or diarrhea, depression, anxiety, fatigue, hair loss, weight loss and easy bruising. It reportedly affects about 1% of the population, but more and more people are being diagnosed with Celiac disease, especially in aging populations.[28] Currently, there are about 3 million diagnosed with Celiac disease.

Why all the hype? Why should anyone else who doesn't, as far as they know, have Celiac disease, care about gluten being in their food or not?

We should all care because Celiac disease is essentially only one of many gluten-related disorders that the majority of us have without being aware of them.[29,30,31] And, as symptoms of Celiac disease can vary a great deal from patient to patient, a delay in a proper diagnosis is quite common. Many cases of Celiac disease go undiagnosed; it is estimated that only 5 percent of people with Celiac disease know that they have it. Only 3 million have received a formal diagnosis; therefore, that leaves almost 60 million people walking around this country with a potential for Celiac disease who don't know they have it![32]

For some people, constipation is the main symptom, while for others the main symptom is diarrhea. Yet in many others, there is no stool irregularity or other gut issues. Only 1 in 8 people with Celiac disease even have intestinal symptoms.[33]

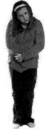

The common "gut" symptoms of Celiac disease include: abdominal pain, gas, bloating, indigestion, a distended stomach, nausea, vomiting, a decrease in appetite, an intolerance to lactose, weight loss that cannot be explained, and stools that float, have blood in them, appear fatty, or are quite foul smelling.

Non-digestive related symptoms include: bruising easily, pain in the joints or bones, depression, children with growth delays, hair loss, fatigue, malnutrition, changes in behavior, anemia, irritability, skin problems, seizures, ulcers in the mouth, decrease in bone density, muscle cramps, swelling, hypoglycemia, nose bleeds, difficulty breathing or catching the breath, defects in tooth enamel or discolorations, and deficiencies in vitamins or minerals such as folate, vitamin K, or iron.

People with Celiac disease have a higher risk of other disorders and diseases as well, and therefore, a myriad of even more non-gut symptoms. They are more likely to have another or other autoimmune disorders such as rheumatoid arthritis (RA), Hashimoto's thyroiditis, systemic lupus erythematosus (SLE), type I diabetes, reproductive disorders and Sjögren's Syndrome. Also, those with Celiac disease have a greater risk of certain types of cancer including intestinal lymphoma and bowel cancer as well as increased risk of disorders of the nervous system—these can include tingling or numbness in the hands and feet (peripheral neuropathy), Alzheimer's, Parkinson's, multiple sclerosis and even seizures.[25,34,35]

Why it's worse than you might think and why you should care

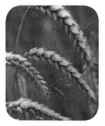 It turns out there are plenty of other reasons to be concerned about gluten.

Let's go back to the statistics. It is estimated that at least 60 million Americans are walking around completely unaware that they have Celiac disease. We know that approximately 3 million people have a confirmed diagnosis of Celiac disease. We also know that all celiac patients have gluten-reactivity, as that is one of the criteria for the diagnosis of Celiac disease.

Okay, so you don't have bowel issues and you are seemingly feeling just fine....and maybe you are likely to be predisposed to a gluten-related disorder. Who cares?

You should, and here's why.

Only a small percentage of those with gluten-reactivity have Celiac disease; less than 1%. It has been estimated by Kenneth Fine, MD, of the Intestinal Health Institute, that upwards of 81% of the population is likely to be predisposed to a gluten-related disorder. We are seeing more and more that the true 'disease' or 'disorder,' despite all of the various diseases we've mentioned thus far, is perhaps only one 'disorder,' gluten-reactivity, and that all of these other named 'diseases' are simply a symptom or manifestation of the prime issue.

Many people have what is now being termed in the current research as "non-celiac gluten sensitivity." This means that the person does not have Celiac disease but is having an immune reaction to gluten. The reaction may be an immune system response but without the classical intestinal enteropathy. There are also other gluten-related disorders that can, with cumulative exposure to gluten, cause chronic disease.[36]

The presence of gluten in foods can lead to an immune reaction in just about anyone, causing inflammation. This inflammation, as stated earlier, eventually results in "leaky gut," or more appropriately termed, "increased intestinal permeability." This condition causes even more immune reactions due to the exposure to other proteins in the food we are digesting – proteins to which the immune system otherwise, if the intestinal lining was fully intact, would not be exposed. These can cause immune reactions to eggs, dairy, and other every day foods such as tuna, apples, green beans, etc.

The already up-regulated immune system begins to get even more stimulated and begins to attack proteins from foods we commonly eat. Food proteins are chains of amino acids. Some sections of these chains are similar to sections of amino acid chains that make up organs, tissues or enzymes, referred to as "self." The immune system can then react more and more against these "self" proteins, damaging not only the intestines but other organs and systems as well.

This gluten-reactivity cascade, which starts as inflammation of the gut, can lead to a multitude of symptoms in the gut itself. If left unchecked or untreated, this can also lead to long term damage of other tissues in the body and present as a multitude of common chronic diseases. This is due partly because of the nutritional deficiencies created by the inflammation of the digestive system, but also from direct attack by the immune system on other organs, tissues and systems, particularly in those with a genetic predisposition to autoimmune disease.

Gluten, whether you have Celiac disease or not, irritates and alters the lining of the gut, resulting in damaging inflammation and what is known as intestinal permeability or 'leaky gut.' I know we may be sounding like a broken record with the leaky gut business, but it is very important that this is understood and appreciated. A leaky gut allows bacterial toxins, viruses and undigested proteins from food, including gluten and the proteins that gluten and other foods break down into, to slip through the gut lining and in some cases enter into the blood stream. The immune system, not normally exposed to these 'invaders' in one with a healthy gut barrier, gets triggered to attack these proteins. Food proteins are now no longer 'food' for the body, but get registered by the immune system as "enemy invaders."[37]

The immune system is programed to differentiate between "self," the tissues, organs, hormones, enzymes, that make up the body and keep it functioning optimally, and non-self-antigens (viruses, chemicals and other toxicants). The problem with gluten, and other substances that begin to leak out of the gut, is that many of these proteins closely resemble, or are almost identical to the 'self' proteins that make up and are used by other tissues in the body, thus stimulating the immune system to begin to wrongly recognize your body as an enemy and attacking it every time you eat certain foods.

Many of these disorders are autoimmune disorders—where your own immune system attacks your own body. And, once you have one autoimmune disease, you are at greater risk for others. Essentially, once the control of the immune system and 'self-tolerance' is lost for one tissue or organ, it increases the chances that the immune system will attack other tissues or organs – especially if the gluten-trigger keeps coming in the foods you eat and the immune system keeps stepping up to attack and you begin to react against transglutaminases, which are an important building block in most body tissues. It has also been shown that transglutaminases may be elevated in various forms of cancers[38,39] and neurodegenerative diseases such as Huntington's disease[40] and Parkinson's disease.[41] Interestingly, transglutaminases are used in the commercial food industry as a binder for processed meats[42]– think imitation crab and processed lunch meats.

Why Wheat is the Scariest of All Grains

First, in order to understand why wheat is so scary, we need to have an overview of required nutrients and how our digestive system gets them into our bodies

Our digestive systems are designed to take the large molecules found in food and systematically break these large molecules down into smaller and smaller particles so that these pieces can be absorbed through the cells that line the intestines, and can be used as nutrients for every cell of our body.

To give you a basic idea of the types of nutrients our bodies are made up of and/or require:

- **Water**—Every cell in your body is "bathing" in water and there's lots of varying advice out there on how much pure water to drink, but a reasonable rule of thumb is 2- 2.5 liters per day or ½ your body weight in ounces every day.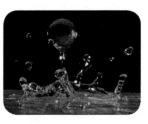

- **Proteins**—Proteins are made up of long chains of substances called amino acids. Some of these are called "Essential Amino Acids" and are required in the diet because our bodies cannot make them. A "complete protein" contains all the essential amino acids. Proteins can be thought of as the "engine" of the cell—they are the main component of enzymes, substances that are essential to speeding up and performing the hundreds of biochemical reactions that occur 24 hours a day, 7 days a week. Other proteins act as structural support—in the muscles for example, proteins provide the scaffolding that allows for the sliding movement of muscles. Other proteins include those that communicate between cells. Proteins also make up our vital organs, muscles, skin, hair and nails.

- **Carbohydrates**—Carbohydrates are made up of chains of various types of sugars. Carbohydrates can be complex or simple sugars—like the sugars you may add to your coffee or tea. Glucose is a simple sugar and so is fructose—the kind that is found in high fructose corn syrup. Although glucose and fructose are both simple sugars, their chemical structure is quite different. The complex carbohydrates are like those you would find in raw grains, fruits and vegetables. The functions of carbohydrates are complex – for example, carbohydrates help store energy and provide the "backbone" of DNA (and remember, our DNA makes up our genes).

- **Fiber**—Necessary for healthy bowel movements, is primarily a carbohydrate which is not absorbed—and therefore stays in your digestive tract to help move things along.
- **Lipids**—Lipids or fats have gotten a "bad name" but are now becoming recognized for their importance in health and nutrition. They are a large class of substances and include the different types of cholesterol, essential fatty acids such as the omega-3 fatty acids and triglycerides, among others. Lipids also can function as energy storage, structural elements of cells, vitamins and signaling substances.

We are warned about high cholesterol levels, for example—but cholesterol is found in every single cell of your body in the cell membrane—and, performs an absolutely vital function in the membrane, allowing the membrane to be flexible. Cholesterol also plays a role in regulating the traffic of what comes into or leaves the cell.

Omega-3 fatty acids are involved in a whole variety of functions— these are the fatty acids you want to increase in your diet. The omega-6 fatty acids perform different functions—but, they are found in so many different foods (while omega-3s are a little bit harder to come by) that in general, we encourage increasing the omega-3 fatty acids and watching the amounts of omega-6 fatty acids we take in. A third type of fatty acid is the omega-9 variety found in olive oil—that type of fatty acid is similar to the omega-3s, so increasing that by using olive oil in your salad dressing is a great idea.

- **Minerals**—We divide the required minerals into two groups—the "macrominerals" and the "trace minerals." We require quite a lot of the macrominerals and much less of the trace minerals. That doesn't mean that the trace minerals aren't important, though! They are! The macrominerals are calcium, sodium, potassium, magnesium, chlorine, phosphorus and sulfur. The trace minerals include, among others, iodine, copper, iron, manganese, selenium and zinc. Minerals perform a wide variety of functions necessary to keep those cellular engines running at their best.

- **Vitamins**—The vitamins can be divided into two main classes, the fat soluble vitamins such as vitamins A, D, E and K and the water soluble vitamins such as the B complex vitamins and vitamin C. The fat soluble vitamins get stored (in fat), but the water soluble vitamins are used and then quickly eliminated in the urine. They perform various important functions…the name "vitamin" is, after all, derived from "vita," Latin for life.

- **Intestinal bacteria and probiotics**— By some estimates, the number of intestinal bacteria is about 10 times the number of human cells![44] These organisms are essential for producing vitamin B12 and vitamin K, for proper digestion, and for "training" certain aspects of our immune systems. These bacteria are symbiotic with us—both benefit from the relationship. It has been estimated that 70% of our immunity comes from these beneficial bacteria.[44,45]

- **Other nutrients**. The list of "other nutrients" is a long one and includes substances like anti-oxidants and bioflavonoids, phytoestrogens, and other nutrients that support and nourish us and are being investigated as anti-inflammatory agents, antibiotics and even anti-cancer agents. These are the types of nutrients you find in fruits, vegetables, tea and berries (anti-oxidants, bioflavonoids), vegetables (phytoestrogens, isothiocyanates) particularly in broccoli, cauliflower and brussel sprouts.

Now, for a quick look at the digestive process:

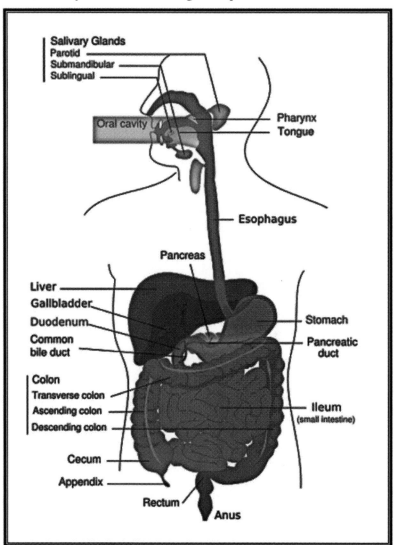

Figure 1: The Digestive System

Digestion starts in the mouth, where enzymes in the saliva start to break down carbohydrates. This is one of the reasons it is important to chew your food at least 31 times. Why 31? Really, because it's an odd number and 31 chews pretty much guarantees the food will be easy to swallow.

After swallowing, the food enters the stomach, where the acids in the stomach start to break down proteins and continues to break up the carbohydrates. The stomach churns and mixes the food (that is the "gurgling" you sometimes feel…and hear!). The food, now called chime, moves into the small intestine, meeting up with bile from the gall bladder (which helps to digest fats) and juices from the pancreas which neutralize the acids from the stomach and contain a number of different enzymes that continue to break up the substances in the food.

Most nutrient absorption takes place in the small intestine—which actually has a really deceptively big surface area—in adults, the small intestines are about 22-23 feet long. To increase the nutrient absorbing area even more, the inner lining of the small intestine has multiple folds in it—and then, on a microscopic level, there are even more folds—this might give you some idea of how important it is to health to properly absorb all the nutrients available in food.

After most of the nutrients from food have been absorbed in the small intestine, the waste passes into the large intestine. One of the main functions of the large intestine is to retain water for the body by reabsorbing water back from the stool. Another function is provided for by the intestinal bacteria—these bacteria produce vitamin B12, vitamin K (necessary for proper blood clotting), biotin and thiamine. The other main function of the large intestine is the storage of feces until elimination by a bowel movement.

Now, back to wheat and gluten, and why wheat in particular is so scary.

Wheat gets broken down (digested) by our digestive system into many different proteins and peptides (the even smaller building-blocks of proteins). Some of the proteins and peptides that are found in the breakdown of wheat include, *the gluten molecules – omega, gamma and alpha gliadins and glutenin - opioid peptides - gluteomorphin and prodynorphin - and a lectin called wheat germ agglutinin.*

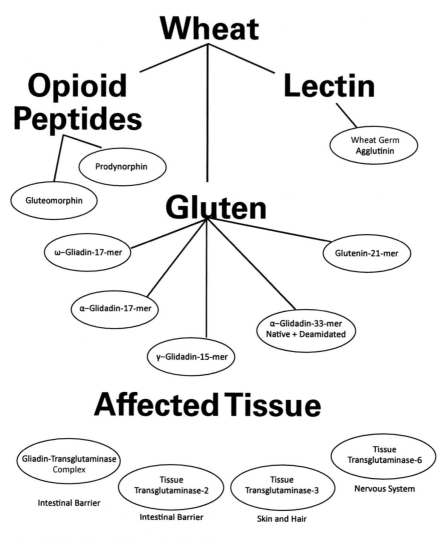

Figure 2: The Breakdown of Wheat and its Affected Tissue

Antibodies to alpha-gliadin-33-mer and tissue transglutaminase-2 (tTG2) are those antibodies that are assessed by most labs testing for Celiac disease. This conventional test is measuring immune reactions to the alpha-gliadin-33-mer protein, which is only one of several gliadins. The others that one could react to: several alpha gliadins, omega gliadin, glutenin, and gluteomorphin.[46] Allergy (IgE response) to omega gliadin has been linked to exercise-induced asthma.[47] There are several documented reports of people experiencing asthma during exercise after eating a meal containing gluten.

What this means, is that common laboratory testing may result in a 'false' negative for gluten-reactivity if one was tested only for reactivity to alpha gliadin-33-mer, which is in fact what most labs test. Therefore, many people who have been tested are walking around potentially thinking they are negative for gluten-reactivity when they could be reacting to a different wheat protein or peptide. Unfortunately, these potentially, and likely, gluten-reactive folks are still consuming deadly gluten-containing foods.

Wheat Germ Agglutinin (WGA) is a lectin protein found in whole wheat. The term "agglutinin" was applied many years ago because it was found that under certain circumstances, it will agglutinate, or clump, red blood cells. In fact, because it binds so well to certain substances, it is often used in research to purify substances such as insulin and red blood cell membranes. If a person reacts to WGA, it can lead to severe reactions and inflammation throughout your body, and is linked

A FEW BRIEF WORDS ABOUT THE IMMUNE SYSTEM.

There are two types of immune responses—the cellular response and the antibody response. The cellular response is based on a variety of immune cells that react to a foreign substance (antigen) by producing substance called cytokines—the cytokines carry on the immune response. Antibodies are proteins that very specifically bind to antigens. These two "arms" of the immune response often work together to produce inflammation or to combat an infection.

There are 5 classes of antibodies—also known as immunoglobulins (Ig's). The most abundant in the blood stream is called IgG. The first antibody that is made in response to an antigen is IgA followed closely by IgM. IgE is part of the allergic response. IgD is an antibody about which very little is known. IgA is the most abundant immunoglobulin in the mucosa that lines exterior surfaces of the body and is found in the gastrointestinal tract mucosa and in tears and the mucosa of the lungs and vagina. It is the first defender against antigens that are ingested or inhaled.

to Celiac disease,[48] diabetes,[49] and other gastrointestinal disorders.[50,51] Once again, with common standard lab testing, this person may have tested 'negative' to 'wheat-reactivity' because only the alpha gliadin-33-mer antibody was tested.

Here's where things get really scary:

As we mentioned earlier, aside from gliadins and agglutinins, wheat is broken down into other substances: glutenin (also from gluten), a sticky glue-like substance that we use to hold baked goods together, gluteomorphin and prodynorphin are also a product of improper wheat digestion. Gluteomorphin and prodynorphin are opioid peptides. Yes, opioid, as in opium, which can affect your brain and nervous system just like the addictive drug after which it is named. Research has shown that these peptides can bind to receptors in the brain interfering with normal brain function.[52] It has also been found that autistic children are very susceptible and sensitive to these peptides. It also might explain the addictive nature of wheat-based products. This is another example of the effect of gluten beyond the gut and intestines.

One can have reactivity and several types of immune reactions to any of these breakdown products of wheat and gluten. The issue is that, depending on which one(s) you are reacting to, your immune system may also be triggered to attack your body's own tissues and chemicals, especially if there is genetic predisposition for this to happen.

You see, transglutaminases, are a family of enzymes that are used by the body in many different tissues to 'bind' proteins together to help create the scaffolding of our barriers and structures and which are therefore required for normal healthy brain function, skin function, bone function, intestinal function and the function of most other tissues, glands and organs.[53] These transglutaminases may link to the proteins and peptides from wheat digestion, travel to where they are exposed to certain immune cells that then react to destroy them. The issue with this is that now your immune system may be triggered to inadvertently destroy your otherwise healthy brain tissue, leading to the common degenerative brain diseases that we all worry about getting: Alzheimer's, Parkinson's, dementia, etc. Your immune system may also be triggered to attack your thyroid, resulting in a disorder known as Hashimoto's thyroiditis; your pancreas, resulting in Type I diabetes; your bone tissue, resulting in osteoporosis; or your joints, resulting in rheumatoid arthritis (RA). This list goes on and on, but you get the picture.

The inflammation and increased intestinal permeability (leakiness) incited by wheat/gluten ingestion can lead to your immune system attacking any one or more different tissue transglutaminases:, Transglutaminase-2, Transglutaminase-3, Transglutaminase-6. We may develop reactivity to these enzymes without even having reactivity to gluten or gliadin, but the message here is clear:

When you have Gluten-Reactivity, every time you eat wheat and other gluten-containing grains you could be attacking and destroying yourself! Every time you eat these foods, you may be killing your body! Every time you eat these foods you may be one step closer to illness, disease and death!

Tissue Transglutaminase-2

Antibodies to Tissue Tranglutaminase-2 (tTG2) are a strong indicator of gastrointestinal autoimmunity. When the test for this antibody is seen positive in addition to that for gliadin antibodies, this becomes a very strong indicator for Celiac disease. If one tests positive to tTG2 but negative for gliadin, then this person may have other autoimmune diseases without having Celiac disease. Because tTG2 is found ubiquitously throughout the body, a positive tTG2 test could mean your immune system is stimulated to attack the intestinal lining (as in Crohn's disease),[54] brain tissue (as in Parkinson's) or skin (dermatitis herpetiformis),[55] etc.

Tissue Transglutaminase-3

Reactions against Tissue Transglutaminase-3 (tTG3), also known as Epidermal Transglutaminase due to its predominance in skin and hair shaft follicles, have been linked with many degenerative diseases and is found to be associated with dermatitis herpetiformis and Celiac disease,[56] Huntington's disease, and because it may 'cross-react' with the other transglutaminases, may also play a role in the diseases associated with tTG2 and tTG6.

Tissue Transglutaminase-6

Here's a biggie. Tissue Transglutaminase-6 (tTG6) is found and expressed in neural tissue. Scientists have found elevated antibodies to tTG6 in the blood of Schizophrenia patients,[57] patients with other neurological and psychological manifestations with or without Celiac disease,[58] autism,[59] cerebral palsy,[60] gluten ataxia,[61] and peripheral neuropathies.[62]

Another scary characteristic of wheat digestion, is the Gliadin-Transglutaminase Complex. In some cases the gliadin protein and the transglutaminase enzyme will bind together forming a new complex. The complex will adhere to the intestinal barrier wall. Our immune system will attack the complex, and in the process destroy the intestinal barrier. This action further increases intestinal permeability. There it is again – Leaky Gut!

A leaky gut and the genetic predisposition for reactions to proteins and peptides from wheat, or for immune and other reactions to other gluten-containing products, then you have the stage set for a "perfect storm." This may at least in part explain why Alzheimer's disease, diabetes, Hashimoto's thyroiditis and other autoimmune-related diseases of the brain and body are on the rise.[63,64]

Part Two:
Gluten Does Not Discriminate

Autoimmune and other diseases

As discussed previously Gluten-Reactivity has been discovered in a significant number of people with severely debilitating autoimmune diseases. Remember, most people with gluten-related disorders do not even have Celiac disease.

This means that even though you may not have Celiac disease or any noticeable bowel symptoms, gluten may be triggering the deadly and silent attack of vital organs and tissues in your body. Over time, this can cause permanent damage, ruining your quality of life or leading to death. And with an estimated 80% or more of the population being reactive to gluten or its by-products, and eating it by the boat-load, for every meal of every day, that likely means this may be happening to you.

We've mentioned classical Celiac disease is the genetic predisposition to gluten reactivity causing an inflammatory reaction in the intestines. Some researchers claim that gluten-related disorders is a group of diseases itself; diseases that may involve several organs outside of the intestines and without Celiac disease, resulting in Type I diabetes,[65,66] multiple sclerosis,[67,68] systemic lupus erythematous (SLE),[69,70,71] autoimmune thyroid disease,[72] rheumatoid arthritis,[73,74] Addison's disease,[75,76] vasculitis,[77] autism,[59] asthma,[78] neurological disorders and seizures,[79,80,81] Alzheimer's and dementia mimicking gluten ataxia,[82,83] Parkinson's,[84,85] dermatitis herpetiformis (a rare skin disease) and other skin conditions such as psoriasis and psoriatic arthritis,[86,87,88,89] headaches,[90,91] liver disease,[92,93] cancer,[94,95,96] muscle disease/myopathy,[97,98] depression,[99,100,101] and likely many other autoimmune and non-autoimmune diseases once thought to be independent of each other. Research is demonstrating more and more that THE underlying disease may be a gluten-reactivity.

Diabetes and gluten

UnitedHealth Group's Center for Health Reform and Modernization predicts that by 2020, more than 50% of the population of the U.S. will have type 2 diabetes or pre-diabetes. Gluten may very well be part of the issue, especially for those folks who have diligently worked to eliminate the obvious sources of elevated blood sugars such as soda and candy.

Many of the patients that we see in our office are working to reverse their type 2 diabetes. We run the most sophisticated gluten-reactivity testing currently available for our patients. Even before this laboratory opened up, when we could only test for the alpha-gliadin-33-mer antibody we found the majority of our type 2 diabetic patients were reacting to gluten.

Moreover, these folks often also expressed the signs and symptoms of autoimmunity and autoimmune disease. These disorders include some of those already mentioned, as well as some others: Hashimoto's thyroiditis, gout, rheumatoid arthritis, lupus, scleroderma, celiac, etc.

Not only are most of the type 2 diabetics that we see reacting to their food, but they are also showing signs of the autoimmune process—their immune systems are attacking their own body tissues. Many of them also suffer from significant signs of brain degeneration (Alzheimer's, gluten ataxia, etc.).

If you are eating gluten-filled foods throughout the day, which is likely the case, if you are eating the Standard American Diet (SAD), AND if you have gluten-reactivity, which according to our research is more than likely, you are, in essence, causing your body to attack this 'enemy,' and inadvertently destroying tissues and organs in your own body. This is "collateral damage" at its most personal level!

The resulting immune system inflammation causes your body to try to handle the damaging effects (pain, swelling, tissue damage) by producing its own 'anti-inflammatory agent.' This natural anti-inflammatory is called cortisol, and it is derived from the adrenal glands that sit atop each of your kidneys. Cortisol acts in the body similar to anti-inflammatory drugs. Anti-inflammatory drugs include cortisone and prednisone.

Cortisol causes the body to shut down insulin receptors and to release sugar out of storage and into the blood stream. Sometimes, this is a good thing and is needed. But, if it is stimulated to be released day in and day out, meal after meal, hour after hour, because of the ingestion of gluten and the ensuing inflammatory response that is created, then your body will be creating elevated blood sugars. This is a source of frustration for our patients who have cut sugars out of the diet, but continue to see high blood sugars and the need for multiple diabetes medications. Their body is generating high blood sugars as a secondary response to the inflammation caused in the body by eating gluten!

Feeling a Little Stress?

Chronic stress happens to all of us and is defined as a continuous, long-term condition where the stress that you perceive is at a constant, unremitting level. It's important to remember sometimes that stress means different things to different people—and, even if you don't think you are under stress…well, your adrenal glands just might have a different idea.

Certain hormones and substances are produced when anyone believing they are in danger or perceive themselves to be under stress—or their body perceives itself to be under stress. The two main hormones are cortisol and adrenaline. This is part of the "Fight or Flight" response. Those hormones and substances can give someone enough energy to fight—or enough energy to run away, maybe climb a tree – any response necessary to get out of the situation fast. Another important thing to remember is that our "Fight or Flight" response has been evolved over thousands of years, to allow us to get away from a dangerous animal, situation or person. But—and this is an important BUT…it was not designed to deal with constant stress—the type of constant stress that many of us deal with on a daily basis. The adrenal response evolved to protect us against the occasional emergency situation.

Cortisol is controlled very closely by what is called the HPA (Hypothalamic-Pituitary-Adrenal) axis. The hypothalamus secretes a hormone CRH (Corticotropin Releasing Hormone) that in turn, causes the pituitary to secrete ACTH (AdrenoCorticoTrophic Hormone). ACTH is then secreted into the blood and acts on the adrenal glands to secrete more cortisol and adrenaline. Cortisol and adrenaline work together to make sure there is enough energy to either "fight" or "take off in flight" by increasing the amount of blood sugar and oxygen in the body. Blood sugar is one of the main fuels and oxygen helps us "burn" that fuel. Other organs and systems respond as well. When cortisol and adrenaline are released:

- Blood flow is channeled away from less vital organs to vital organs, like the brain, the heart, the lungs and skeletal muscle (those muscles that will help you fight....or climb a tree to get away from the danger).
- The heart rate and blood pressure increases to pump more blood to the vital organs faster.
- Breathing rate increases to get more oxygen to the tissues.
- The liver is signaled to break down its stored blood sugar to provide instant useable energy.
- Other organs and tissues produce more sugars and release the sugars into the bloodstream.

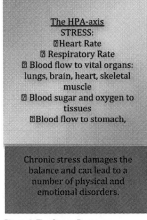

The HPA-axis
STRESS:
⬆Heart Rate
⬆ Respiratory Rate
⬆ Blood flow to vital organs: lungs, brain, heart, skeletal muscle
⬆ Blood sugar and oxygen to tissues
⬇Blood flow to stomach,

Chronic stress damages the balance and can lead to a number of physical and emotional disorders.

Figure 3: The Stress Response

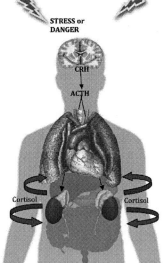

STRESS or DANGER
CRH
ACTH
Cortisol
Cortisol

All of these responses are normal – and can be very useful, when it happens in a real emergency. So why is chronic stress bad for you?

As mentioned, this is a normal physiological response, meant to be only temporary—just to get you out of an emergency situation that happens occasionally. But, if like many people, you have constant—chronic—stress in your life, the body responds by adjusting over and over again, trying to keep up—and we –or our adrenal glands—just get exhausted. Then, when another stressful situation occurs, the body simply has nothing left to give. This can lead to all sorts of problems, both in physical and mental health.

For example, a recent paper linked Metabolic Syndrome, often considered a pre-diabetic condition, with chronic stress. People with chronic stress were twice as likely to have Metabolic Syndrome as those without stress. Metabolic Syndrome is a condition of high blood pressure, high blood glucose and lipids, low HDL cholesterol and abdominal obesity. Chronic stress also puts you at risk for heart disease, obesity, stroke, diabetes, high blood pressure and other conditions. Chronic stress affects you emotionally as well, leading to depression, anxiety, a loss of ability to concentrate and memory problems.[102,103]

There are other problems caused by constant stress and cortisol release as well. Cortisol is produced in a diurnal, or a 24-hour cycle. Cortisol is the hormone that works in a healthy body in opposition with melatonin to regulate your sleep/wake cycles. It is a stimulatory hormone that helps to wake you up in the morning. It also happens to work in the body to stimulate the release of sugar that is stored in your liver and muscles into the blood stream and to inhibit insulin receptors in order to keep sugar in the blood stream.

When you are causing continuous inflammation due to constant exposure and reactions to gluten and grains, the adrenal glands perceive this as stress—and you are relentlessly driving your adrenal glands to spit out cortisol, not just in the morning to wake you up, but all day. In many cases, the push goes all night too in an attempt to inhibit the damage caused by the inflammation and to put out the fires caused by your immune response.

This is the same thing that happens when you take prednisone or cortisone (orally or by injection) to get inflammation down. Some of our patients tell us they became diabetic soon after commencing a course of treatment with oral steroids.

If you are a type 2 diabetic who turns out to be positive for a gluten-related disorder, then you must fully eliminate that trigger from your diet in order to reduce the inflammation in your body, and ultimately reduce the negative effects of elevated cortisol on the body. This is a common source of insulin resistance for type 2 diabetics (one of many).

Why Grain-free for a diabetic is even better than Gluten-free

Many of our diabetic patients do very well when cutting out gluten-containing grains from their diets. We take things a step further and have them completely (especially initially) eliminate all grains from the diet. The rationale for this is four-fold.

First, as discussed before, when we cut out all grains, we are sure to eliminate gluten, which reduces inflammation and helps to bring down sugars and weight.

Second, and of utmost importance for a diabetic, all grains contain difficult to digest proteins, proteins that the immune system may confuse with gluten thus causing an inflammatory response. They may all lead to nutritional deficiencies if eaten in excess.

Third, all grains contain significant amounts of sugar, which whether gluten-free or not, will likely cause blood sugar to spike and further contribute to and worsen their diabetes.

Fourth, grains contain significant amounts of omega-6 fats, which when consumed in excess, and without equal amounts of omega-3 fats, increase inflammation, which then contributes to diabetes, heart disease and cancers.

If that's not reason enough to get checked for gluten-reactivity, or to simply eliminate it completely, we don't know what is.

Hashimoto's Thyroiditis and Gluten

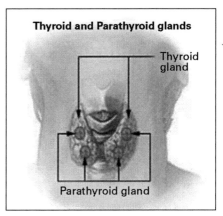

Thyroid and Parathyroid glands

Thyroid gland

Parathyroid gland

Figure 4: The thyroid and parathyroid gland

The thyroid gland plays a central role in maintaining energy levels, temperature, weight, clear thinking, the sensitivity of the body to other hormones and the synthesis of proteins. (See Figure 4) It is located at the base of the neck and wraps around the front of the neck. There are two conditions that affect the thyroid:

- Hypothyroidism (an UNDER-active thyroid)
- Hyperthyroid (an OVER-active thyroid)

The most common form of hypothyroidism is Hashimoto's thyroiditis. This is an autoimmune disorder where the body is producing antibodies against the thyroid and therefore attacks the thyroid. It manifests as periods of hyperthyroidism followed by periods of hypothyroidism as the thyroid is attacked and then goes into remission. Eventually the continuous destruction of the thyroid leads to the decreased production of thyroid hormones and chronic hypothryoidism. It is estimated that 90% of hypothyroid cases are Hashimoto's autoimmune thyroiditis.[104]

The most common cause of hyperthyroidism is Graves' disease—this is also an autoimmune disorder, but in Graves' disease, the antibodies stimulate and increase thyroid hormone production and you get too much.

Some Hashimoto's cases occur after or during pregnancy, after viral or bacterial infections, or after long periods of stress.[105] Both hypo- and hyper-thyroid occurs predominantly in women starting at the ages of 30-40. Some cases of Graves' disease have been associated with exposures to heavy metals[106] and prescription drugs.[107]

T4 and T3 are the main thyroid hormones. T4 is also known as "thyroxine" and T3 is known as "triiodothyronine". The numbers 4 and 3 represent the number of iodine atoms per molecule of hormone. Iodine is a critical nutrient for the proper functioning of the thyroid gland. In the body, T4 is converted to the active T3 form. T3 then enters just about each and every cell of our body to help regulate temperature and overall metabolism—the sum of all the biochemical reactions that go on in our bodies. Because of this role in metabolism, T3 is critical to the proper use of proteins, fats, vitamins and carbohydrates in the body. T3 also is important for the development and maintenance of the brain and nervous systems, the overall hormonal (endocrine) systems and our response to stress.

Thyroid specialists have noticed that a significant number of patients with Hashimoto's thyroiditis and Grave's disease also have gluten-related disorders or have Celiac disease. An average 2-4% of all patients have both an autoimmune thyroid disorder and a gluten-related disorder. Recent reviews have suggested that physicians check their patients with thyroid disease for gluten-related disorders and Celiac disease—and that physicians check their patients with Celiac disease or gluten-related disorders for thyroid disease.[108,109]

The connection and mechanism between Hashimoto's and gluten-reactivity has been discussed previously, but it is very important to understand that the main trigger for the immune system to flare up and attack the thyroid is exposure/ingestion of gluten. Every time that a person with Hashimoto's eats gluten, the immune system is stimulated to attack the thyroid. It is not as simple as just taking your Synthroid™ or thyroid supplements and thinking that the problem with your thyroid is handled. It is understanding what causes the immune system to attack and that every time your system attacks your thyroid, you have less and less thyroid left, and thus become more and more hypothyroid as time goes by, and ultimately need higher and higher doses of medications to compensate.

There are many other triggers for the autoimmune destruction of the thyroid, but we have focused on the main one, gluten, since this book is about gluten and its role in almost every disease.

It is also important to understand, if you suffer from hypothyroidism (and are thus likely to have Hashimoto's based on the statistical odds), that there is a higher incidence of thyroid cancer in the Hashimoto's population.[110,111,112] Thus, it stands to reason that doing all you can to avoid the main trigger for the thyroid inflammation, gluten, would then help also decrease your odds of thyroid cancer.

Autism and Gluten

Gluten-reactivity has also been found to be a significant issue in children with autism.[59,113]

Autism is a disorder that is a major concern amongst parents, pediatricians, and educators. It is widely recognized to be a growing problem in this country and around the world. Because this disorder is becoming more common each year, rising at a rate of 15% each year, it has sparked a great deal of debate and research into the reason behind its development for treatment purposes.[114,115, 116]

Although autism is being looked at from many vantage points with regards to what causes it and what perpetuates it, new studies, especially those that have been based in the alternative medicine field, have found that there is a potentially strong link between food reactivity and autism, especially a link between gluten and the condition. This new data suggests that gluten may create reactions and immune responses that either cause (directly or indirectly) or worsen autism. We do know that autism and autism spectrum disorders are multi-factorial and are influenced by genetics, environment and diet.[60]

Autism is a disorder that affects children's cognitive development and cognitive function. This can cause problems with communication abilities, behavior, and social interaction. While it was thought that autism may be genetic, recent studies have found that environmental factors may actually be the cause of, or influencing trigger for the disorder. It is likely that certain external (environmental) factors can trigger a hidden genetic potential for this, and any disease, which may explain the ever increasing rates of autism as well as autoimmune diseases.

Research is beginning to reveal that mothers of autistic children are more likely to be autoimmune themselves (often unknowingly) and that many of these mothers have antibodies directed to the cerebellum and brain of the developing fetus (this is proof of the immune system's attack on that tissue). We don't entirely understand why most of the time, a mother does NOT develop antibodies to her developing fetus. Part of the fetus' genetics is the mother's—or "self," so it is not as likely to elicit an immune response. But, the other part of the fetus' genetic background comes from the father—and from the mother's point of view, is "non-self" and should elicit an immune response. The fact is, however, for most pregnancies, the mother's immune system accepts the fetus. It is thought, however, if the mother already has a predilection for autoimmune responses, her system may react to the fetus—and this may produce the antibodies to brain tissue mentioned above.

While more research is certainly needed, it seems likely that at least one factor in what we believe is a multifactorial condition is that the autistic child's brain development is affected in the uterus by maternal antibodies. It is thought that these antibodies cross the blood brain barrier and cause inflammation in the brain of the developing fetus. This may lead to abnormalities in brain function and may result in triggering the child's own autoimmune disease tendencies[117,118,119] The autistic child is more likely to suffer from autoimmune conditions such as Celiac disease and food reactivity, particularly to gluten and other common cross-reactive proteins such as those found in dairy.[120,121,122,123,124] The autistic child has a higher prevalence for having autoimmunity to other tissues, in particular brain and cerebellar tissues, which may explain in part the neurological and behavioral issues associated with autism.[32,33] This means that a female with Hashimoto's, or any autoimmune disease triggered by gluten, eating gluten during the pregnancy may flare up her immune system to attack, resulting in the simultaneous attack of not just her own tissues, but those of her unborn baby, resulting in the infant having autoimmune diseases and/or a greater chance of developing autism.

To make matters even worse, the autistic child is susceptible to conditions such as "leaky gut" and "leaky brain." This makes the child more at risk for further immune responses to other proteins besides gluten.

And it gets more complicated, because that child's immune system is also responding to break-down products of gluten and other proteins. Studies that have tracked autistic children with gluten-reactivity have found that gluten is broken down into small proteins known as exorphins, or opioid peptides. These peptides behave much like morphine and related opiates would. And, with the "leaky gut" and "leaky brain," these substances enter the child's body and travel to the brain where they attach to opioid receptors. When opioid receptors are 'clogged' by opioid peptides, brain messaging chemicals called neurotransmitters cannot send their signals for neurological function.[125] This may explain the heightened state of psycho-sensitivity and aberrant behaviors (hyperactivity, OCD, unusual and repetitive motions) often seen in autistic children. This also explains why the simple step of the elimination of gluten from the autistic child's diet often results in improved function at all levels and fewer 'outbursts.' Since immune responses to gluten can affect the whole body of an individual sensitive to it, causing a variety of mental and physical symptoms, it is not unreasonable to suspect that the consequences for a child with autism and sensitivity to gluten can be incredibly debilitating and far reaching.

"Brain fog" is considered to be a mental symptom of autism, but it can also often be mistaken for other psychiatric conditions including depression, anxiety and even more serious conditions. And, as much as we don't always want to admit it, just how many of us have 'brain fog' at least occasionally? Many people have it MORE than occasionally and are walking around in a perpetual fog and don't even know it. After all, you have to BE aware in order to know that you are NOT aware! It's a mental Catch-22 situation. So, gluten, while being a trigger for neurological issues for anyone with gluten-reactivity, is particularly profound in its effect on one with autism due to the existing neurological inflammation with the resulting behaviors.

Gluten-reactive adults are often plagued by the more obvious physical symptoms resulting from consuming gluten containing foods. Children, especially autistic children, tend to suffer more from the cognitive and behavioral side effects, such as brain fog, concentration issues, depression, moodiness, behavior issues or difficulty with socialization skills. If these children are never "screened" for gluten-related disorders, or no one ever thinks to check their diets, these children will likely be put on multiple medications to "control" their behavior and the simple, straightforward approach of dietary control will never be properly investigated.

Just as the remedy for a gluten-reactive adult is a gluten-free diet, parents with children showing symptoms of mental impairment, behavioral issues, learning struggles and lack of focus may want to consider eliminating gluten from the daily diet as a first line of therapy before resorting to having the child take any medication.[127]

Many parents have added casein-free diets as well. Casein is a protein found in dairy products and the rationale for the removal of casein from the diet is similar to that of gluten. Many parents report positive changes in their children after a period of time (usually at least over 2-3 months, sometimes sooner, sometimes later). And, while the criticism is often made that there are few clinical studies proving the benefits of a Gluten-Free Casein-Free (GFCF) diet and parent's reports are "unreliable," it should be admitted that parent's reports seem to be reasonably reliable when a doctor wants to put a child on multiple medications—what reason is there to not respect the same parent's reports when a simple dietary intervention is put into place?

There have been only a few clinical studies regarding a Gluten-Free Casein-Free (GFCF) diet.[126] In one study, 10 pairs of children were compared after a full year of a GFCF diet. The pairs of children were randomized and the results were evaluated by blinded observers— meaning that some of the most important aspects of a well-run study were used. Another positive aspect to this study was that it went on for a full year, allowing for a wide range of responses to the GFCF diet. The results were positive and significant. In the children on the GFCF diet, social contact increased in 10 of 15 of them. Ritualistic or repeated behaviors decreased in 8 out of 11 of the treated children.[127]

Another study looked at potential benefits of a casein-free diet—in this study, children with autism had improvement in their behavioral symptoms after 8 weeks on a dairy elimination diet.[128] Other studies have used various methods, but overall, the results have been promising.[129] Interestingly, many of the studies have concerned potential nutritional deficiencies for children on the GFCF diet.[72,73,130,131] The concerns are primarily with the B vitamins and iron—and it is really important, by the way, to ensure that everyone on a GFCF diet do get enough of these important nutrients.

The best food sources of the B-vitamins are meat, poultry and fish, as well as leafy green vegetables such as spinach, chard, mustard greens, kales and other vegetables such as broccoli, green beans and asparagus. Legumes such as black beans and lentils are also a great source of the B vitamins. Vitamin B12 is found in high levels in organ meats such as liver, as well as in poultry, fish and other seafood. Iron can be found in high levels in artichoke, parsley, spinach, broccoli, green beans, tomato juice, tofu and other soy products, seafood and beef liver. An interesting thing to realize is that fewer studies seem to be concerned with the effects of the medications commonly used on these children's nutrition, growth and development, than with the "safety" of the GFCF diet.

The truth is that eating grains (with or without gluten), increases malabsorption of vitamins and minerals in general. Therefore, avoiding the consumption of all grains helps improve the absorption of vitamins and minerals from animal, fish and vegetable and fruit sources.[101]

If your child has been diagnosed with autism—or even if he or she hasn't, but you suspect that food reactivity is playing a detrimental role in the health of your child, there are a number of things to keep in mind.

- You should be patient, because it can take as long as 6 to 9 months before the inflammation caused by gluten, casein and any other food intolerance calms down enough to let the body heal, and allow for changes in behavior and physical/mental symptoms to become clear.
- You may need specific nutrients (vitamin supplements) to heal the damage, so seek professional medical guidance if necessary.
- Ensure that the diet has sufficient vitamins and minerals, particularly

paying attention to the B-vitamins, iron and the Essential Fatty Acids (EFAs), the omega-3 fatty acids.

In her book, <u>Louder Than Words</u>, actress Jenny McCarthy talks about her son Evan, his diagnosis with autism and her search for answers. Jenny implemented a gluten-free diet (along with medication, therapy and supplements) to help Evan battle the effects caused by autism with positive results.

Attention Deficit-Hyperactivity Disorder (ADD/ADHD) and Gluten

ADD and ADHD are the most common behavioral disorders diagnosed in children. About 3-5% of kids carry this diagnosis (some would say "label"). Like autism, it is more often diagnosed in boys than it is in girls.

The symptoms experienced by these children generally fall into one of three groups:

- A lack of attention: this can include difficulties in staying focused, paying attention to directions, an apparent lack of listening skills, difficulty in organizing activities, appears absent-minded, often losing track of toys, school assignments, books and being easily distracted.
- Impulsive behavior: this can include a difficulty in taking their turn, interrupting, difficulty in anger management, blurting out responses.
- Hyperactivity: this can include fidgeting, repetitive behavior, an inability to play alone or quietly, constantly changing positions, excessive talking and inappropriate running or climbing.

Children may fall into one of these groups, or may have some characteristics from each group of symptoms. Technically, to be diagnosed with ADD/ADHD (and many children are mis-diagnosed), the kids need to show either 6 attention symptoms or 6 impulsivity/hyperactivity symptoms in more than one setting before the age of 7. Other potential causes need to be excluded and these symptoms need to be severe enough to cause difficulties in a number of settings—home, school, play-groups, etc. Many of these children are on combinations of medications and go through behavioral therapies as well. The list of medications used for ADD/ADHD include:

- Amphetamine-dextroamphetamine (Adderall)
- Dexmethylphenidate (Focalin)
- Dextroamphetamine (Dexedrine, Dextrostat)
- Lisdexamfetamine (Vyvanse)
- Methylphenidate (Ritalin, Concerta, Metadate, Daytrana)[132]

Some doctors treating children with ADD/ADHD will try elimination diets – eliminating gluten and/or casein, sugar, food additives and colorants.[133] Many children have benefited from these elimination diets.[34,135,136,137] The best-known of these diets is the Feingold diet, which removes additives and foods which contain salicylates, a substance similar to aspirin, which can stimulate the dis-regulated immune system to attack. The elimination of gluten, casein, sugar and food additives can be challenging but is well worth it to improve behavior without risking the side effects of medication.

From Mild Depression To Schizophrenia

So maybe you don't have autism or ADD/ADHD, but maybe you suffer from mild to moderate depression. If so, this could also be related to gluten-reactivity. If it is, you will definitely want to consider eliminating gluten from your diet.

If you have depression, or any mental condition causing you to feel moody or blue, if you choose NOT to address this with the simple step of eliminating gluten, this, in fact, could lead to major problems down the road. Your symptoms of mild depression, irritability, anxiety, agitation or other issues with mood may indicate that gluten is affecting your body as a whole, including your brain, and may in fact be an early warning sign of diseases to come. Seasonal Affective Disorder (SAD) may also be an early warning sign that gluten is causing widespread yet subtle damage and destruction to your brain.

Research is continuing to try to find the connection between gluten-related disorders and mental issues and disease, ranging from depression and anxiety to Seasonal Affective Disorder, and bipolar disorder and all the way to schizophrenia. One study confirmed and concluded that schizophrenia is associated with gluten-reactivity[138] and that symptoms of schizophrenia abated with the elimination of gluten from the diet and flared up with re-exposure to gluten.[139]

Gluten-reactivity was described in one study as a systemic autoimmune disease with diverse manifestations and that many individuals without Celiac disease manifest solely with neurological dysfunction.[26]

One practicing pediatric gastroenterologist (a specialist in children's digestive disorders), Rodney Ford, MD, has stated in an article that gluten causes brain disease. He states that he came to that conclusion after studying the effects of gluten on his patients for more than a decade. He theorizes that the brain is the common pathway for the manifestations of all gluten symptoms.

This sensitivity of the brain to gluten may explain other neurological manifestations that many of our patients describe, particularly our diabetics; depression, loss of balance and coordination, gait changes, mental fatigue, brain fog, memory loss, Alzheimer's, Parkinson's, and multiple sclerosis.

An association between gluten and nerve tissue damage has also been shown in those with multiple sclerosis.[21] Researchers are now recommending that doctors test MS patients for Celiac disease, gluten sensitivity or for gliadin/gluten antibodies and putting these patients on a gluten-free diet.[44,47,140]

Gluten Ataxia

As mentioned, one of the other very important systems besides digestive system that is adversely affected by gluten-reactivity is the neurological (nervous) system. There are many possible symptoms including developmental delays and learning disorders in children, depression, migraine, and headache in both children and adults. And remember that gluten-related disorders and Celiac disease are both under-diagnosed. So, this reactivity can result in autism, ADD/ADHD, depression and outright psychoic disorders. But muscular control can be affected as well.

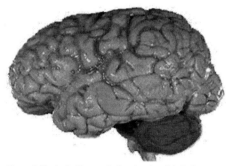

Figure 5: The brain *(the cerebellum is colored darker)*

One of the most common effects on the nervous system in gluten-reactivity is known as cerebellar ataxia. The cerebellum, colored darker in Figure 5, plays an important role in the control of movement such as talking, walking, reaching and running. Ataxia can be defined as a "sudden, uncoordinated muscle movement due to disease or injury to the cerebellum in the brain."[141] Symptoms can involve areas of the body from the neck to the hips, the arms or the legs. These movements can be seen as a sudden side-to-side motion or a back and forth motion. These movements can also make a person look like their arms and legs are swaying. Speech can be affected as well—so a person with cerebellar ataxia can have slurred or awkward speech, problems with walking, and/or repetitive or uncontrolled eye movements. This type of movement disorder is actually sometimes called "gluten ataxia."[142] Early treatment by removing gluten from the diet most often leads to great improvement, if the cause is gluten and will often completely stop the progression of the neurological damage.[85]

We mentioned that wheat and gluten breaks down into smaller proteins. Some of these proteins are opioid peptides which may act essentially like opiate drugs (morphine). We also know that our body's own enzymes (transglutaminases) may get bound up with gliadin and other wheat-based peptides, causing our immune systems to attack. Transgutaminases are used in the brain. Some people develop an immune response to tranglutaminase-6, if left unaddressed, this immune response could result in an attack on the tissues of the brain (in this case the cerebellum).[37,38,41,143]

This means that every time a gluten-reactive person with antibodies to certain tissue transglutaminases eats wheat bread, they may trigger their immune system to attack their brain. And—they likely don't even know that this is what is happening.

We have had several patients describe how, after beginning to eat a gluten-free diet, the balance and gait issues they had for years that they attributed to getting older, cleared up within a few days. One patient spent years waking up and staggering around the house as he states, "Like I was drunk." After only one week off grains and gluten-containing foods, he started waking up and walking around alert and with a completely normal gait. Another interesting thing that this patient in particular noted was that his long-term and short-term memory was slowly returning on this new diet. Clearly, he was destroying his brain every day that he ate oatmeal, cereal, pasta, bread and the like. He was suffering daily brain degeneration by autoimmune attacks brought on every time they ate gluten-containing foods. Damage to the brain was caused by exposure to grain!

Peripheral Neuropathy

Another common neurological problem seen with gluten-reactivity is called peripheral neuropathy. Peripheral neuropathy (PN) most often affects the hands and feet. It is usually described as feelings of numbness, pain or tingling along with a possible loss of sensations such as touch or sensitivity to vibration or temperature. It is often referred to as a "stocking and glove" neuropathy because some people will describe a burning and others may describe the loss of sensation, feeling like they are wearing socks or gloves.

Now, there are many causes of peripheral neuropathy—it can be caused by injuries, infections with viruses or bacteria, exposure to various toxins (such as gluten), and by other conditions such as diabetes. But, it is quite often seen in people with gluten-reactivity and Celiac disease as well. The connection between all of these is the "alerted" immune system causing damage to the peripheral (outer) nerves of the hands and feet.

The most common type of PN in people with gluten-reactivity involves both sensations and movements. Many people don't realize at first that there is a problem—they think they are clumsy or absent-minded. Not feeling the differences between hot and cold, not feeling vibrations and not knowing how well you are holding on to, say, a cup of tea may be the first symptom. A sense of "clumsiness" or a feeling as if you don't know where your feet are or where your arms are may be another. Movement may be affected as well but may first be noticed as increased tripping or falling.

In fact, there are some researchers who believe that Celiac disease (CD) and gluten-related disorders (GRD) are more neurological disorders than immunological ones and should be treated that way. In a recent article in the journal Medical Hypotheses, the author suggested that both CD and GRD should be considered a neurological disorder because the neurological symptoms can show up in people without any intestinal damage or intestinal symptoms.[144] These authors suggested that the neurological damage may occur before intestinal damage is there and without any intestinal symptoms.

Osteoporosis

Two other conditions –for both men and women—that are associated with gluten-related disorders and/or Celiac disease are osteoporosis (thinning and weakening of the bones) and osteopenia (lower than normal bone density).

Bones go through a continuous process of forming and re-forming. This growth and remodeling slows down to some degree as we age. Also, as we age, the bones can become osteoporotic or osteopenic. There are genetic (family history), hormonal, as well as environmental, and nutritional factors that can be important. It's a long list, but that list includes gluten-related disorders and Celiac disease as well as hereditary disorders, endocrine disorders, chronic disease and cancers. Some of the other risk factors that may be important include decreased physical activity, steroid use (for example prednisone for more than 3 months), Vitamin D and/or vitamin K deficiency, or a deficiency in calcium and phosphorus, heavy alcohol use, a family history of osteoporosis, having a white or an Asian ethnic background, low body weight and a history of smoking.

Osteoporosis and osteopenia can be silent-- there are few early warning symptoms. Later in the disease, a person can experience bone pain or tenderness. This pain can often show up in the neck or low back. Most commonly, the first sign of bone disease is a fracture or break at the wrist or femur (below the hip), or in the bones of the spine, the vertebrae. One of the well-known leading causes of osteoporosis is the drop in estrogen that accompanies menopause, though it is important to remember that men are at risk for osteoporosis as well. In fact, there have been some patients who were diagnosed with previously unknown GRD or Celiac disease because their complaints of muscle weakness and bone pain, which turned out to be osteoporosis secondary to nutritional deficiencies that have been associated with GRD/Celiac disease.[145,146]

The main problem that is putting people with gluten-related disorders or Celiac disease at risk for osteoporosis and osteopenia appears to be a problem of getting adequate levels of calcium and vitamin D, as well as other nutrients.[147] There may, however, be additional factors.

It may be that gluten-reactivity damages the digestive system such that calcium and Vitamin D are poorly absorbed, setting up a disorder known as secondary hyperparathyroidism.[148,149] The term secondary is used because the first problem was GRD/Celiac disease and the parathyroid condition was the second problem—and it is the second problem that is directly related to the development of osteoporosis.

The parathyroid glands are located on the thyroid gland, found at the base of the neck. The thyroid gland controls a great deal of your energy and metabolism—all the biochemical reactions going on in every cell of your body. The parathyroid glands are four small areas on the back side of the thyroid—these glands regulate calcium (Ca), phosphorus (P) and vitamin D. They are about the size of a grain of rice and secrete a hormone named parathyroid hormone (PTH) or sometimes parathormone. The main role of PTH is to keep the body's calcium levels within a very narrow range—too much or too little calcium in the blood and tissues can seriously affect your health, particularly your heart, skeletal muscle and your nervous system. When the calcium levels drop below a certain level, the parathyroid gland begins to produce and secrete PTH. PTH then increases the calcium levels in the blood by stimulating calcium release from the bones, which are essentially a storage bin for calcium. At the same time, PTH will increase calcium absorption from foods and slow down kidney excretion of calcium. Vitamin D production begins in the skin with exposure to sunlight and the presence of cholesterol, and is required to make calcium-binding proteins that allow for this increased absorption from foods. As the calcium levels in the blood increase, the phosphorus levels (in the form of phosphates) decrease—so as the calcium goes up, the phosphates are reduced. While phosphates don't directly affect the secretion of PTH, diets high in phosphates, such as high soda and grain diets can cause increased secretion of PTH.

Calcium (and phosphates) is essentially stored in the bones. So, if a long-term calcium deficiency exists because of dietary deficiencies or malabsorption because of long-term gluten-reactivity, the parathyroid gland may become overactive—grabbing more and more calcium from the bones to keep blood levels of calcium within a normal range. A vitamin D deficiency worsens the problem. The eventual result may be osteoporosis.

In a recent study of 255 postmenopausal women with osteoporosis but without any signs or suspicion of gluten-related disorders, almost 10% were positive for serum anti-gliadin antibodies and positive for tissue transglutaminase antibodies—they were gluten-reactive but had no symptoms.[150] In another study, individuals with osteoporosis were found to be 10 times more likely to have intestinal damage due to gluten-reactivity.[151] This suggests a number of things—that gluten-related disorders and Celiac disease are under-diagnosed in postmenopausal women, and in patients being treated for osteoporosis, and that underlying gluten reactivity may be a root cause of bone disease.[152]

Once again, as stated earlier, a direct assault on bone tissue, or bone building substances may occur if the immune system is triggered by gluten proteins to attack the bone itself.[153]

A third trigger for bone thinning is that chronic inflammation (possibly triggered by gluten) results in the constant release of cortisol (our body's anti-inflammatory). Constant exposure to cortisol results in the thinning of bone tissue (as in the case of prednisone or cortisone use).[154,155]

Based on the most current research findings, it seems very clear that at least for a significant number of people, gluten and its derivatives are immune system dis-regulators and neurotoxins that can lead to the immune destruction of your brain and nerve tissue and almost ANY other tissue or organ of the body. One of the biggest problems here is that most people are totally unaware of the threat. They may go from doctor to doctor, be put on medication after medication—and never find out that the problem may be in that sandwich they have for lunch every day.

In essence, if you suffer from, are concerned about, or have a family history of: diabetes, hypothyroid disease, multiple sclerosis, lupus, rheumatoid arthritis, heart disease and stroke, Celiac disease, migraines and headaches, seasonal allergies, gout, Alzheimer's, Parkinson's, Crohn's, ADD/ADHD, irritable bowel syndrome, dementia, depression, cancer, liver disease, infertility, psoriasis, eczema, asthma, depression, constipation, diarrhea, anemia, fibromyalgia, osteoporosis, polycystic ovary syndrome, vasculitis, or chronic fatigue, then you should eliminate gluten-containing foods and cross-reactive foods from your life completely and forever.

Patients in our office are screened for gluten, all of its breakdown proteins as well as all of the cross-reactive foods their body may be reacting to and/or confusing for gluten, and true to the predictions, approximately 80% of folks who walk through our doors with any myriad of 'diseases' are reacting to gluten.

A Gluten-free diet and weight loss

If you Google the phrase "gluten-free weight loss", you get over 5 and a half MILLION hits! Now, that doesn't exactly constitute proof—but is there a real relationship between going on a gluten- and grain-free diet and weight loss?

Well, yes and no, there are two sides to this answer. We have discussed Celiac disease and many of the common symptoms from which patients with this condition suffer. One of the common symptoms used to help diagnose Celiac disease is weight loss. This is primarily because of the malabsorption and malnorishment caused by the inflammatory process of the disease. So when a person that has Celiac disease starts a gluten-free or grain-free diet many times they notice weight gain. And this is a positive sign, their body is healthier as a result of this diet change and their body is able to metabolize the nutrients they are consuming.

Now on the other hand, we have non-celiac gluten-sensitive individuals that many times exhibit a different result. There is not a great deal of research on this yet, but we have seen the results clinically, experienced by many patients—and, there's a rationale for weight loss when going gluten-free. Humans have been evolutionarily designed to store excess carbohydrates (and fats) as fat tissue. When you decrease the carbohydrates and inflammation by eliminating gluten and grains in your diet (taking care, of course to make sure you have enough protein, fiber, vitamins and minerals—and the healthy fats), those who are underweight tend to gain weight while those who are overweight, lose it.[156,157] The carbohydrates in grains tend to cause a spike in blood sugar—with the complex carbohydrates, that spike is slower than with simple carbohydrates.

The body responds to increased blood sugar by secreting insulin— and one of the things insulin does is it lowers the levels of blood sugar by increasing the storage of excess sugars as fat tissue. If you eat high carbohydrate/sugar meals a good deal of the time, the levels of insulin get high and a number of damaging things happen. First, your cells can get insulin resistant—and this is a precursor to the condition, diabetes. Also, consistently high insulin levels can suppress other hormones that are needed to burn up the excess fats and sugars that the body has stored.

First of all, when you go gluten-free you change the types of carbohydrates you eat. The carbohydrates in vegetables, fruits, beans, and seeds are complex carbohydrates of a different chemistry and in lower amounts than are found in grains.

Second, these foods contain different proteins that do not cause inflammation as readily as those found in grains. Vegetable, nuts and fruits are a good source of dietary sugars that do not contains highly inflammatory proteins such as gluten to fire up your immune system, which can result in an attack on your body.

Third, if you follow our plan, eating smaller, grain-free meals and snacks with only about 2-3 hours between eating, the spikes in blood sugar do not occur and the amount of insulin secreted is less- so there is less likelihood of developing insulin resistance, a condition that most often leads to obesity, heart disease and diabetes. And, since spikes in blood sugar are lower and allow for more of the sugars to be used as energy right away (as opposed to being stored as fat), you can begin to use those ....ummmm....storage areas...more efficiently because the lower levels of insulin allow the release of the other hormones that are responsible for burning up the stored fat as energy (glucagon and growth hormone).

Fourth, as you start feeling better and more energetic you naturally become more active, and that's when you can begin to lose even more weight. Let's face it, when you are overweight and feeling awful, it's not the most efficient or potentially most successful time to start exercising.

One way to think about the foods you should be eating is to eat like your ancestors did. Remember, grains were only domesticated about 10,000 years ago—that was the agricultural revolution that began, we believe, the rise of towns and cities. But, on an evolutionary time scale, that is a very short time. In other words, humans evolved eating foods that were not grains—and 10, 000 years is not enough time for humans to have developed the ability to digest those grains very efficiently. For some people, this is not an obvious problem—at least they don't have symptoms. But they may have symptoms in the form of obesity. For others, depending on their particular genetics, it is not simply obesity, but one or more of the diseases listed in previous chapters.

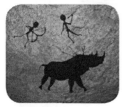

Genetics play an important role in the development of obesity, though it is not yet clear which genes are involved and in what combinations.[158] There are clearly other factors involved – genetics and family history alone can't explain the fact that the obesity rate in the US has doubled in the last twenty years.[159] Other factors include increased availability of high calorie, processed foods and decreased levels of physical activity and exercise. Another major factor is the grains that we eat.

Also, the concept of the "thrifty gene" has been proposed to explain the increases in the rates of obesity. The "thrifty gene" is a gene (or genes) that would be useful in times of famine or the low availability of food—if there was no food available, those people who carried a gene that increased the storage of fat as a source of energy could come in quite handy—and those people would survive to pass that gene down to their children. But, when there is lots of food available, as there is for many in the US, that thrifty gene is instead, a liability.

Think of weight as an energy balance. Because of our evolutionary history (particularly before the domestication of grains) our bodies are geared towards protecting against too little energy (a negative energy balance). The way we protect ourselves from too little energy and too little food is to store it as fat whenever we can. Grains provide the carbohydrates which can be stored as energy. Most modern people, on the other hand have too much food, and burn too little calories to justify even eating grains anymore. So, our bodies do what hundreds of thousands of years of experience indicate is a smart idea—store that energy in the form of fat for those times when food is short. If you begin to eat like your ancestors did, then you can begin to tip the balance back and just provide yourself with the energy and nutrition you need and not encourage your body to store energy as fat. And, our ancestors did not eat grain.

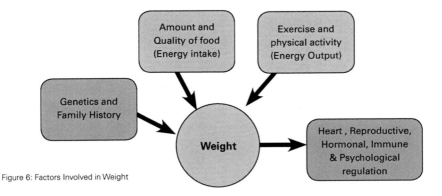

Figure 6: Factors Involved in Weight

How do I know if I have a gluten-related disorder?

Most labs, as discussed previously, test for only one of several gliadins. Based on the fact that wheat breaks down into a multitude of proteins and peptides that may cause a negative reaction in your body, you can see just how limiting some conventional testing is. Many people test 'negative' for 'gluten-reactivity,' meaning they were only tested for alpha-gliadin-33-mer, yet may still be gluten-reactive because there are several other gluten proteins from wheat to which you could be reacting.

When we test with the more specific testing, rarely done in the current standard testing model, we find more people reacting to gluten and suffering from gluten-related disorders. This means that for some unsuspecting individuals, their form of immune reaction to the breakdown products of wheat/gluten is an indication of likely autoimmunity that may lead to Hashimoto's Thyroiditis, Type I diabetes (insulin dependent) and/or brain diseases (Alzheimer's, gluten ataxia, multiple sclerosis, etc.). If you've noticed lately that you are forgetting where you put your keys, are losing balance and tripping or dropping things more than usual, this could be you and you should get a comprehensive test for gluten-related conditions and autoimmunity. We primarily use Cyrex Labs to test for gluten-related disorders and autoimmunity. This lab has a number of different tests using blood or saliva to specifically test for gluten-reactivity and autoimmunity. Visit our website: MyLivingHealth.com or TheSkinnyDocs.com for more information on testing.

To make matters even more complex, most labs that test for gluten (alpha-gliadin-33-mer) reactivity, test for only one type of immune reaction, a specific antibody immune response called IgA. This is done as the routine 'gluten' test by most labs because the positive result for IgA for alpha-gliadin-33-mer is a needed result to confirm Celiac disease. The problem is that only a small percentage of people who have gluten-related disorders have Celiac disease. There is a greater portion of the population that has non-celiac gluten sensitivity/reactivity. This group likely may not test positive for this one gliadin molecule or that specific type of immunoglobulin. In fact, researchers have shown that 50% of celiacs do not make antibodies to alpha-gliadin-33-mer.[160] IgA is the immune response most abundantly found in mucus or mucus producing tissues/glands (for example, producing saliva), while IgG is the response most abundant in blood/serum immunity.

Cyrex labs, the company we use for testing, uses patent pending testing that offers comprehensive panels that assess both common delayed immune responses (IgA and IgG) to various wheat proteins, peptides and biomarkers of gluten-related autoimmunity. This gives us the most reliable way to determine to what a patient is reacting, and how this impacts a patient with regards to:

- What to eat?
- Are there risks for autoimmunity?
- What elements to include in or exclude from a personalized nutrition plan?

The answers to these questions help us to calm and "reset" the patient's immune response, reverse disease progress and achieve optimal health goals.

Cross-Reactivity – Yikes!

Now that we have fully covered the multiple proteins and peptides of wheat and gluten, let's move on to another "OMG!" concept. Gluten proteins, specifically alpha-gliadin-33-mer, can cross-react to other foods. What is food cross-reactivity? Just like the autoimmune process we discussed earlier, the amino acid chain that makes up the gluten protein, alpha-gliadin-33-mer, can have similar sequences to the amino acid chains of other food proteins. When your immune system is not functioning properly, the antibodies programmed to detect alpha-gliadin-33-mer may, for example, mistake whey protein from cow's milk as alpha-gliadin-33-mer. Thus, the gluten inflammatory response continues even though the patient is on a gluten-free diet.

Many times we find patients that have gone the gluten-free diet route, still complain of many, if not all of the same symptoms. As a result, for many folks, when they eat and digest other common 'healthy' foods, even gluten-free grains, their immune system mistakes these substances for gluten or gluten derivatives. This unfortunate error results in immune reactions to proteins that are found in foods generally considered 'gluten-free'.

We find that there are a couple of different reasons for continued discomforts. One reason mentioned above is the similarity in the structure and therefore the immune system cannot distinguish the difference between the two – cross-reactivity. Another reason may be the consumption of foods unaccustomed to the digestive system – lack of tolerance. During infancy the human immune system learns that food proteins are good and therefore the immune system should not react to them. The immune system develops "tolerance" to those foods exposed to the infant in the first few years of life. If by going gluten-free, you simply substitute regular, gluten-filled breads, cookies and crackers for gluten-free versions, you expose yourself to many grains that were not introduced to you when you were a baby. As a result, the immune system may react negatively to the newly-introduced foods. Yet another problem we see with patients starting a gluten-free diet, is that they over consume certain gluten-free foods. They think anything labeled "gluten-free" is ok. This over consumption of gluten-free items can create or stimulate new reactivity. Finally, patients may believe they are being gluten-free, but in fact are consuming 'hidden' sources of gluten in their diet or through their health and beauty products.

Yikes!

This is how we assess the gluten-free diet:

GLUTEN-CONTAINING GRAINS To uncover hidden exposures to gluten	Rye, Barley, Polish Wheat, Spelt
CROSS-REACTIVE FOODS	Cow's Milk, Casein, Milk Butyrophilin, Casomorphin, Whey Protein, Chocolate (milk), Oats (wheat-contaminated), Yeast, Coffee
NEWLY-INTRODUCED FOODS	Sesame, Buckwheat, Sorghum, Millet, Hemp, Amaranth, Quinoa, Tapioca, Teff
OVER-CONSUMED FOODS	Corn, Rice, Potato
COMMON FOOD ALLERGENS	Soy, Egg

Therefore, in order to really know if a gluten-free food is safe for you to eat without making you sick, you need to know to which of the above foods you react and don't react. Visit our website: MyLivingHealth.com or TheSkinnyDocs.com for more information about testing.

The safest bet is to simply make the leap into eating grain-free for life. By going grain-free you will eliminate the majority of the potential trouble sources. This may initially sound crazy, extreme, or just plain impossible, but we can tell you from our personal experience, and after working with thousands of patients, that not only is it possible, but very likely how we as humans were intended to eat and did eat for millions of years until recently.

This is the future of health care. As individuals we are each similar but we are also very unique. We see this every day demonstrated by the test results from patients in our office. We may see test results from ten diabetics, these patients are similar because they suffer from high blood sugar, but the results from the gluten-reactivity and gluten-associated cross-reactive tests are very different and unique. One may show signs of gluten, hemp, buckwheat and potato reactivity while the next shows signs of gluten, yeast, oat and soy reactivity. The cookie cutter diet plan would not be effective for these individuals. In order to get results a customized dietary plan must be designed for each of them.

Part Three:
Living a Gluten-Free Life

What is it Like Going Gluten-Free?

John's Story

John came to our office because he was tired of his health declining despite taking multiple medications, and being treated by several doctors. John was extremely selective in his choice of physician and had sought some of the top doctors in their respective fields.

John was 66 years old and had been diagnosed with type 2 diabetes and high cholesterol. We sat with John and discussed his prior treatments, medications and his goals. During our consultation John described feeling dizzy, light headed and off balance for the first couple of hours after waking in the morning. This was a fairly new sensation but one that was of great concern.

We did a series of tests on John to determine what was causing his conditions and to determine a treatment plan. One of the tests we did on John was a stool test, which among other things, tests for the alpha-gliadin-33-mer antibody reaction to gluten and wheat. Then we also ran a saliva test. One part of the saliva test also looks at the alpha-gliadin-33-mer antibody. Both of these test results came back negative, meaning John was not alpha-gliadin-33-mer intolerant or sensitive. In other words, based on these two tests it looked like John was not experiencing gluten-reactivity. If we had stopped testing at this point, we would have missed a significant piece of the puzzle. Upon further testing, which included the blood test that we referred to in the earlier chapter, John tested positive for multiple gluten breakdown products. The Wheat/Gluten Proteome Sensitivity and Autoimmunity blood tests were positive! He was reacting to multiple subproducts of wheat/gluten but not the alpha-gliadin-33-mer product. That is why it is so important to test more than just the alpha-gliadin-33-mer antibody which is the typical test performed to check for gluten-reactivity.

We began working with John on multiple lifestyle changes, one of which was the elimination of gluten from his diet. First we had to educate him on what gluten was and what foods contain gluten. Then we put him on a gluten-free diet, as well as eliminating other gluten-free grains that John was reacting to. The results have been nothing short of amazing. A couple of weeks after making the change John noticed that when he got up in the morning he no longer felt dizzy, light-headed or off balance. We were able to use the Cyrex testing to show that John was stimulating an immune response against his brain and nervous system and this attack was causing his gluten ataxia. This could have led to much more severe health issues down the road, like Alzheimer's and dementia. John has also noticed his memory improve along with his energy levels. He has decreased his medications and has lost weight as well. He is also committed to staying gluten-free.

Now what? How do I go gluten-free without starving?

One of the simplest things that you can do, even without the expense of getting tested, is to go gluten-free and/or grain-free for 7 days and see how you feel. If you notice any positive changes, even as seemingly benign as the feeling of having more energy, or that you can think a little more clearly, then this is a likely indication that you have issues with gluten.

Remember, gluten could be triggering your immune system to attack brain tissue, so this apparently benign issue of brain fog (which we normally excuse as "I guess I'm just getting older" or "I've got too much on my mind—of course I forget a few things!") may be a first clue and an early sign of the dangers yet to come.

The most important tip for someone who is going to cut gluten-containing foods from their diet is to remember that if you take something out, you must put something in its place. You should be full and satisfied after every meal and you should not have cravings throughout the day.

Interestingly, when our patients change to this type of eating plan, they don't have cravings anymore. Previously these patients had reported having all sorts of cravings-- particularly for sweets and junk food. It's an odd but true statement that we seem to crave the foods that are most harmful to our health!

You also need to adhere to a regular schedule of meals and snacks so that you are eating something every 2-3 hours. Many of our patients did not snack. Some skipped meals. This can lead to hunger and intense cravings for sugar and gluten-containing foods. This habit can also lead to metabolic imbalances, weight gain, insulin resistance and eventually type 2 diabetes. If you snack or have some small amount of gluten-free food every 2-3 hours, you will find it much less mentally and emotionally challenging to remain gluten-free or grain-free.

Think of it this way—if you waited to re-fill your gas tank until you were driving on fumes, that would increase the chances of you running out of gas—and it's not the best or most efficient way to drive. In a similar way, you want to eat small amounts of food so that your energy supply—the gas—is always there. Also, don't forget that we sometimes overdo the eating when we get too hungry—or grab the nearest, most convenient food available. And in this society, that often means a doughnut, a bag of chips or some other unhealthy food. This causes the rollercoaster ups and downs of blood sugar and insulin levels. This is a recipe for disease and the eventual use of medication.

We believe, based on years of clinical practice, that the ideal diet is to go completely grain-free, even avoiding the gluten-free options that are now offered on most grocery store shelves. This is a good idea for two reasons:

First, as a general rule, grain-containing packaged foods, regardless of whether they are gluten-free or not, contain sugar. Sugar contributes to obesity, heart disease, inflammation and diabetes, and even Alzheimer's.

Second, remember 'cross-reactivity?' Many foods that are considered gluten-free contain or are digested down into proteins that are similar in structure to gluten. That means that if you have positive immune reaction to a gluten breakdown protein that is similar in structure to that found in, dairy, yeast or coffee, you may also have that same immune response when you eat those foods. When you look at the ingredient list of many of the gluten-free products that are available, they contain a number of the foods that may be 'cross-reactive' with gluten breakdown substances.

Once again, there is currently only one lab (Cyrex Labs) that we know of that performs the tests for this through a panel that assesses foods common to the gluten-free diet, including known cross-reactors:

Cow's milk and it's breakdown proteins, chocolate (milk), sesame, hemp, rye, barley, polish wheat, buckwheat, sorghum, millet, spelt, amaranth, quinoa, yeast, tapioca, oats, coffee, corn, rice, potato, teff, soy, egg.

If a patient in our office doesn't think they can live grain-free for life, then we will run this test to determine what they possibly can eat. If a patient goes grain-free for a period and is perfectly content to do so for life, then there's no need for us to run this test. What a helpful tool, however, to determine if you are not only gluten-reactive, but also intolerant to common foods that are marketed as 'safe' for those who are gluten-reactive.

Generally, if you are not able to go completely grain-free, then the foods to avoid are:

Wheat and all wheat-containing products, spelt, barley, rye and oats. Grains that are generally considered gluten-free and safe for most people to eat are rice, corn, millet, quinoa, and buckwheat. Other food ingredients that are used to make common gluten-free foods, especially baked goods, include: tapioca, potato starch, hemp seed and nut flours.

To complicate matters slightly, there is something else you need to know. It is critical when you go gluten-free to also be aware that monosodium glutamate (MSG) is a problem for many who need to be gluten-free. The unfortunate issue with MSG is that it can be listed on labels by many other names other than MSG. (see Appendix E). This means that foods containing one or more of these items may be a problem for gluten-reactive individuals and will also need to be avoided. Some of these items will list ingredients such as "natural flavor" or "spices." This includes commercial salad dressing, sauces and soups, chewing gum, crackers, chips and most snack foods, even bullion and organic broth may contain hidden gluten. The recommendation by the Food and Agricultural organization of the United Nations and World Health Organizations, which most countries follow, is that foods may contain up to 0.3% protein from gluten containing grains and still be labeled "gluten-free." So read those labels carefully and look for any suspicious ingredients.

A WORD (OR TWO) ABOUT SKIN AND SKIN PRODUCTS

Our skin is one of our largest organs—really. It is the main barrier to the environment but it can let certain substances in and release others. The skin is an organ that many people think is 'waterproof' or impervious to external substances. This is not true, and in fact we have patients apply one or more supplements in cream form for skin delivery. That means that anything you put on the skin is likely to be at least partially absorbed into the bloodstream and circulate throughout the body, for better or worse. When people go gluten-free, they should also consider 'external foods' such as toothpaste, lotion, sunblock, shampoo and conditioner, and cosmetics. A common ingredient in shampoo and conditioner, used as a binder and 'glue' is hydrolyzed wheat, a gluten-containing compound. That means, not only might you be eating gluten, but you might be literally bathing and moisturizing with gluten—it would be as if you are wearing gluten!

When you have decided to go gluten- and grain-free, and go tearing through your pantry, refrigerator and other areas looking for gluten-containing products to get rid of here is a list of items to look at and examine the ingredients:

- Ketchup, mustard and all condiments (even soy sauce is processed with wheat)
- Soups and broths (even organic, which implies pesticide-free, not gluten-free)
- Salad dressing and sauces
- All baked goods, including bread, crackers, muffins, English muffins, pancake and waffle mixes, cookies, etc.
- Cereals and granola's
- Pasta (all shapes and sizes) and pasta dinner kits
- Seasonings: particularly dry-rubs, barbeque seasoning and spice mixes.
- Candy bars, chips and gum and all 'snack' foods
- Dips (humus, chip dip, cheese dips, etc.)
- Rice mixes (dry or frozen pre-mixed).
- Shampoo, conditioner, lotions, cosmetics and toothpaste.
- Seasoned or flavored anything (including bottled drinks and mixes), even if it says 'natural flavors.'

As you can see, this is a pretty extensive list. If you are truly committed to going gluten-free, while it is best to go all out and cold turkey, your budget may only allow you to replace food items over time as they are used up. Do whatever is in your ability to do, and as quickly, and as fully, as you are able. The goal is to be completely gluten-free, since any small amount of gluten can cause an immune reaction and spell damage and destruction for whatever tissue or organ or gland it attacks.

The safe foods include:

- Vegetables
- Meats, poultry and fish (unprocessed)
- Fruits
- Eggs
- Nuts and seeds
- Beans and legumes
- Oils
- Herbs and spices (single spices, no mixes with mystery ingredients)

We recommend that you search for truly gluten-free foods at your local health food store or grocery store and cross-check the ingredients to the lists provided in Appendix D to ensure that they are gluten-free. You can find gluten-free broths, soups, sauces and dressings.

When that's not possible, you will need to make them at home from scratch. This may take some practice in the beginning, as does any new activity, but over time, this will become second nature to you—there is even a chance you will enjoy this new "hobby". Often, when you start making your own dressings, they taste so good, that you really don't have a desire to eat commercial dressings again.

> **MEDICATIONS AND VITAMINS**
>
> You can find a list of gluten-containing medications and vitamins (Yes, medications and vitamins also may contain gluten!) on several websites. But these lists are continually changing and need updating. So the best way to know if your medication or vitamin contains gluten is to ask the pharmacist or contact the manufacturer of the product. Some medications (i.e. synthetic thyroid medication) has gluten in all doses except for the 50 mcg dose, so if you need to be on medication, then you can ask to have your prescription written in the gluten/filler-free dose and take the number required to be at the correct dosage for you.

I know what you're thinking, "If I take out all of the grain, what's left on my plate?" It's simple... Really! We have our patients follow (as we do ourselves), what we have come to refer to as "Dr. Steph's Plate Rule©." One of the common fears of those who are considering going gluten-free or grain-free is what to eat for breakfast, since most of what America eats for breakfast is some form of grain. Dr. Steph's Plate Rule© helps you learn how to eat without being hungry, get all the nutrients you need from your food, lose weight and reverse and prevent disease.

Dr. Steph's Plate Rule©

It all starts with your meals. All meals, including breakfast, should consist of 25% good quality meat, poultry or fish. This works out to roughly 3-6 oz if you are eating on a standard 8-9 inch plate. This leaves the remaining 75% to be vegetables, of which up to 25% of your plate roughly 0-1/3 cup) can be a starchy vegetable, such as beet, carrot, squash, sweet potato, etc.

The remainder of your plate (50-75%) will be unlimited amounts of vegetables that are what we call the 'sticks and leaves.' This unlimited list of veggies includes broccoli, asparagus, lettuce, spinach, kale, chard, cabbage, sprouts, mushrooms, cucumber, zucchini, celery, onions, etc. (see Appendix D for a full list of foods in each food category). This is one of the ways that you fill up, and stay happy and healthy.

Dr. Steph's Plate Rule°

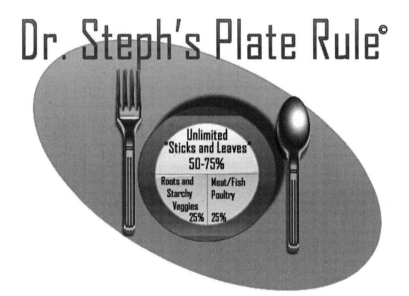

The other way that you will fill up and stay happy and healthy is to consume liberal amounts of healthy oils, including olive oil, macadamia nut oil and coconut oil. Olive oil is an excellent oil to use in salad dressings, and can be poured liberally over your veggies when steamed, baked, grilled, or in salad form. We also use oils in home-made dipping sauces for our meat and fish. Consuming adequate amounts of fat ensures good vitamin absorption, continued healthy structure and function of your brain, immune system, and all cells in the body. And – fats are the primary food that triggers you to feel satisfied and full after your meal.

Fish oil is recommended as a daily food supplement. The brand that we use and recommend to our patients is emulsified and has many co-factors in it so that it is easily digested and absorbed into the body. Coconut oil is recommended for cooking, or can also be taken as a supplement. We recommend anywhere from 2 tsp to 2 Tbsp per day depending on the health conditions with which we are working.

When consuming any oils, you want to get the best quality. That generally means organic, first cold pressed and extra virgin.

What should I have for breakfast?

As stated before, even breakfast should follow the Plate Rule as much as possible. There is no law that prohibits you from eating lunch and dinner foods for breakfast. However, this seems to be a challenge for many people who are conditioned to eating cereal, oatmeal, toast and the like for their first meal of the day. As such, you can find some great products in the grocery store, or online, for breakfast appropriate meats, poultry and fish that you can cook up and eat with veggies. For example, you can find gluten-free, MSG-free, nitrate-free turkey or beef bacon, salmon, beef, turkey or chicken sausage which you can cook up in bulk (great also for evening snacks) and eat for breakfast with steamed spinach, sautéed peppers, onions and mushrooms, etc.

Or you can do what we do and eat leftover hamburger patties with a small salad or on a lettuce 'bun.'

What about snacks?

Snacks are where you put your fruit, nuts and beans, as well as gluten-free grains (if you are keeping those in your diet). You may also eat unlimited amounts of the "sticks and leaves" veggies as well as small servings of meat, fish, or poultry. See Appendix D for recommendations on serving sizes.

Examples of Snacks:
- Sliced apple or pear with raw almond or cashew butter
- Blueberries and raw walnuts

- Cherries and raw almonds
- Celery and carrot sticks with raw nut butter
- Celery sticks or lettuce leaves with tuna salad, turkey salad, chicken salad or salmon salad
- Veggie sticks or Taro chips with humus, bean dip, guacamole

Remember to drink about ½ your body weight in ounces in water every day to keep your system flushing out any residual toxins and inflammatory by-products. This is very important and will help to keep you feeling full—as a side benefit, it will also help keep your skin younger looking!

Scheduling

Your schedule is critical. When do you usually wake up in the morning? You should eat breakfast within 30-60 minutes of waking up. Since you should be eating every 2-3 hours, we recommend that 2 hours or so after breakfast you eat a snack, followed 2 hours after that by lunch and so on and so forth through the entire day.

For example, if you woke up at 7:30, you would eat breakfast at 8:00, a snack at 10:00, lunch around noon, an afternoon snack at 3:00, dinner at 6:00 and possibly a final evening snack around 9:00. This schedule should be kept no matter where you are; at work, at home, running errands, on vacation, etc. It takes some practice planning your days in the beginning, but after some time, you develop new habits that won't easily be broken. You are probably thinking "If I eat that much I'm going to get fat." Actually we find that the opposite happens, you lose weight. This way of thinking is the calories in/calories out theory that was perpetuated in the 70's and 80's. This theory has since been proven false but unfortunately it's still taught and followed by many. The quality of the calories that you take in is a key component in how the body uses them. Do the calories cause a blood sugar and insulin spike and cause you to store fat? Or are they keeping your blood sugar and insulin levels stable helping to keep your body efficiently using the food for energy. The bottom line is the quality is more important than the quantity.

Grocery Shopping Tips

The grocery store can be an intimidating place for a person who is going gluten-free. In order to get the most out of your shopping trip, yet ensure your food choices are completely safe, it is best to approach the store by sections.

Let's begin by taking a virtual trip around the grocery store to highlight the safest areas for gluten-free shoppers.

PRODUCE

The first stop in most grocery stores is the produce section. This section is completely safe, so you should spend a good amount of time here. Make sure you choose a variety of fresh produce, with a range of colors. Choose dark leafy greens, reds, and even purples for your diet. This is also the area that you want to stock up on fruits. Choose berries, apples, peaches, oranges, depending on the season.

Remember to shop for organic produce as often as you can—if possible, shop at local farmer's markets for the freshest, organic foods. Check out the Environmental Working Group's "Dirty Dozen"-those foods that contain the highest levels of pesticides and other chemicals, and the "Clean 15"-those foods that contain the lowest levels of pesticides. Organic foods can be a bit more expensive, so these lists may help you with some of those choices. The most important things to remember about organic foods are that they contain no pesticides AND contain more nutrients than non-organic foods. The reasons for the greater nutritional value of organic foods has to do with the type of farming that organic farmers do—they have to use techniques such as crop rotation and use natural fertilizers to produce their crops. The result is foods with a greater nutritional value.[161,162]

DAIRY

After the produce section, it is time to move on to the dairy section. Most items found in this department are considered to be gluten-free. Just be mindful of the fact that for many folks dairy commonly cross-reacts to gluten proteins. Again, this means that if you are gluten-reactive (or suspect that you are), you should consider avoiding all dairy products as well. Dairy includes butter, cottage cheese, cheese, milk, ice-cream, yogurt, sour cream, cream, and any food product that has milk or milk-derived products in it.

You can opt for milk alternatives, such as rice milk, almond milk, hemp seed milk or coconut milk. Coconut yogurt, coconut butter, coconut oil and coconut ice-cream may also be good dairy replacements. "Fat-free" foods can contain gluten-containing additives and sugars to make the product appear thicker and to taste better, so avoiding these foods is a safer bet.

MEAT/FISH/POULTRY

The next stop is the meat section. Since meat, poultry, and fish are excellent sources of vitamins, minerals, good fats, and protein, you should be sure to choose a nice selection of items. A few suggestions when choosing your protein: when selecting fish choose wild-caught, beef, lamb and other red meats should be grass-fed/grass-finished, and poultry and eggs should be free-range and antibiotic/hormone-free.

We order our meats and fish from several farms in the U.S. that provide the best quality foods in this category. The meat, fish and poultry comes frozen to your doorstep. We have a stand-up freezer in our garage that is regularly stocked with a shelf of beef, a shelf of wild fish, a shelf of free-range poultry, etc. Once a week, we simply pull out a week's worth of food from the freezer, put it in the fridge and whatever is thawed first is what gets cooked a la Dr. Steph's Plate Rule© each night for dinner. See Appendix B for a list of where we order our wild fish and grass-fed meats.

The items you need to steer clear of are prepared, pre-coated, or marinated foods. Or, you will need to check the ingredients list for gluten and MSG. You can find deli meats that are gluten-free, MSG-free, nitrate-free and antibiotic-free, even at most major grocery stores. Once you've taken the extra time initially to determine which products are safe, then grocery shopping becomes a cinch—so much easier than maybe you thought it might be!

BAKED GOODS

As you navigate your way around the perimeter of the store you will find the bakery is usually the next stop. Just keep on walking, since most products here are off limits! This also includes the center aisles of crackers, cakes and cookies, unless you can find 'gluten-free' and have no cross-reactions to the other ingredients, such as tapioca starch, potato starch, rice, quinoa, buckwheat, etc.

Again, we generally encourage a completely grain-free life; however, gluten-free baked goods are a viable option for some people, especially those who cannot imagine life without grains.

For example, some that do okay with rice as a gluten-free food can eat rice crackers, rice cakes, breads and waffles made with rice flour. A word of caution from what we have observed in patients. Make sure you do not go crazy with gluten-free grains. They should be consumed on occasion, not daily. If you have a hard time disciplining yourself then maybe you should consider eliminating grains. This is due to the negative impact they have on sugars.

You can also start looking for 'safe' flours with which to do your own home baking. These flours include almond, rice, buckwheat, coconut, amaranth, millet and even bean flour. Check out the recipe section (later in the book) to find some gluten-free flour mixes that you can easily make on your own. Also look for our recipes for yummy gluten-free treats that don't have any grains at all – and you would never know it!

SAUCES, SOUPS AND DRESSINGS

The majority of your grocery shopping will be around the perimeter of the store. The interior aisles of the store generally contain more junk and gluten-filled food, which will adversely affect your health. Aside from the above-mentioned baked

If you bring your list of MSG/gluten ingredients and cross check this list with the ingredients in many of these products, you will quickly begin to realize why so many people have issues now with gluten, and why America is so sick and overweight – it's in almost everything!

goods, the center aisles are where you will find many bottled, canned and jarred sauces, soups and dressings. Proceed with caution! (Better yet, pass them by with a smile on your face)

Most salad dressings contain gluten as an emulsifier, stabilizer and preservative. Most canned and jarred sauces and soups also contain gluten. What's more, most seasoning packets, rubs and spice mixes contain gluten. Even organic chicken broth will likely contain MSG in the form of autolyzed yeast, which means you will need to specifically seek out gluten-free, MSG-free versions of all of the above, including ketchup, barbecue sauce and soy sauce. They do exist and you will, with persistence, find them and once you do, you're good to go.

FROZEN

The frozen food section can be a bit daunting. Here you should stick to plain fruits, vegetables, beans, and meat/fish items. Avoid products with sauces, seasonings, or coatings, as this is generally where gluten and MSG is lurking. Occasionally, you can find gluten-free turkey or chicken sausage, burgers and bacon. Some companies are even making gluten-free chicken tenders and fish sticks. Again, these are often a safe bet, unless you cross-react with the gluten-free grain ingredients, such as rice or tapioca starch.

The freezer section is where you will also find most gluten-free baked goods such as breads, bagels, English muffins, pizza dough, etc. Once again, proceed with caution. If you have these at all, they should be occasional treats and not part of your everyday meal or snack.

CANNED AND DRIED FOODS

The canned food aisles are safe for the most part IF you stick to single-ingredient foods. While we always recommend fresh veggies and fruits, it is good to know that canned vegetable, fruits, beans, and juices are all safe with regards to gluten. As stated earlier, canned soups should be avoided as they are often thickened with wheat or flavored with MSG. There are other issues with canned food. For example, the cans are lined with a potential carcinogenic plastic that can leach into the food, especially a food that has a high acid content, such as tomatoes. Using tomatoes from a jar is the better option.

Dried beans are the better choice over canned, and are easy to prepare. Simply soak your beans over-night in a container of water, then drain, rinse and simmer in fresh water on the stove until soft. We like to do this in large batches and freeze much of the beans in 2 cup glass dishes for use each week in meals and baked goods (beans make excellent flour replacements in brownie recipes-see the recipe section).

SPICES AND HERBS

This section is easy when you understand what to look for. Any single ingredient herb (dried or fresh), is gluten-free. Any herb/spice mix that contains autolyzed yeast, hydrolyzed wheat, or the mysterious 'spices' should be avoided. Make your own spice and herb mixes. We've included an excellent Taco seasoning mix that takes no time to make, and doesn't contain MSG, which is in most commercial taco seasoning packets. If you make taco meat with this mix, you can use gluten-free shells, romaine lettuce as a shell, or simply make a taco salad with no grains. We like to crush up Taro chips on our taco salad for added crunch.

That's it! If you stick to this outline and some basic guidelines you will have successfully navigated your way through the grocery store with ease. In time, you will find it will become second nature to select food items that are both safe and nutritious.

Meal Prep Tips

Breakfast

Just as with other diet plans, a good gluten-free diet begins each day with breakfast. Breakfast is the most important meal of the day, and can provide a wide range of health benefits. When you are eating a gluten-free diet, breakfast keeps your appetite and blood sugars even throughout the day, making it easier to avoid cravings.

You should always keep a range of breakfast items on hand at all times so it is never a struggle to put together a nutritious morning meal. Starting the day with a high quality protein such as turkey, chicken or grass-fed beef sets your metabolism for the rest of the day.

Remember that we encourage you to eat as per Dr. Steph's Plate Rule© for all meals, including breakfast. Some great options for the protein portion of your plate include turkey bacon, chicken or turkey sausage, beef bacon or grilled chicken. Fresh fruit, fresh steamed vegetables, frozen fruit, dried fruit, eggs, and gluten-free cereal bars are all great options.

We recommend cooking extra amounts of whatever you make for dinner and eat as left-overs for either breakfast or lunch.

A great way to start the day is with a healthy gluten-free breakfast shake. The ingredients that we like to use include protein powder, almond butter, coconut butter/oil, a piece of banana, frozen berries, liquid vitamins, antioxidants, fish oil and water or coconut milk. Then use a hand mixer to blend and serve. Its quick and its healthy!

Gluten-free cereals, gluten-free waffles, gluten-free muffins are not the best way to start the day, and should be limited, or avoided completely, due to the negative effect they have on your blood sugar levels, energy stability and overall health.

Lunch

Once you have conquered breakfast, you need to devise a plan for lunch.

Because of hectic schedules, it is not always easy to slow down and take time for the perfect lunch. By packing your lunch you will be able to know you are eating safely, eating well, saving time, and even saving money.

A thermos of gluten-free chicken soup and a salad works well as do leftovers from dinner the night before. Romaine or leaf lettuce stuffed with tuna salad (or any meat salad) works well and also follows the Plate Rule.

Make a bottle of olive oil dressing and bring it to work (enough for the week) so that all you have to do is either bring your own salad, or run out to the grocery store to pick up a salad and use your own gluten-free dressing.

Dinner

Dinner will most likely be your largest and most elaborate meal of the day.

The majority of your meal should consist of freshly cooked veggies, or a nice big salad, a lean protein source, starchy vegetables, a la Plate Rule. Get creative with the sauces and dressings that you make. There are many resources online for finding good sauce and dressing recipes that are gluten-free.

Snacks

Snacks also follow Dr. Steph's Plate Rule©. We recommend having lots of variety and easy foods on hand. Cut up a lot of veggies and keep in containers in the fridge to grab and go, pre-pack mini zip-lock baggies with single serving sizes of raw nuts that you can keep on hand. They fit perfectly in your purse, briefcase or in the mini-fridge at work so you never go without snacks, and you don't have to worry about eating too much. Keeping fruit on hand is smart. Make large batches of bean dips and freeze them in 2 cup glass jars allows you to have quick snacks with the veggie sticks or Taro chips.

Of course, you can experiment as much, or as little, as you like, but you should try to incorporate variety to keep boredom from setting in. As long as you make your own meals with gluten-free ingredients that you have stocked in your gluten-free pantry you will find you look better, feel better, and can be proud you are doing something healthy for yourself, and your family.

Mary's Story

Mary came in to see us because she was sick, and tired of feeling sick and tired. She was 69 years old, not taking any medications, but was told by her doctor that she should try to relieve her symptoms with medication. She was not happy with that suggestion and felt that in the long run it would only lead to more problems.

Mary came in because she noticed that she could not lose weight despite trying many diets. She felt that she was 30 lbs overweight and wanted the weight gone. Mary also felt that her energy level could be better. She was working full-time, and wanted to continue to do so, but felt if her energy continued to dwindle then she may have to stop working. This was not something she was happy about, because she loved work and felt it added to the quality of her life. She had also noticed that her memory was not as good as it was in the past. She always knew client's names and this ability started to diminish. This scared Mary because her mother was diagnosed with Alzheimer's and she did not want to go down that same path.

We recommended testing, and scheduled Mary for several tests to see if we could determine the cause of Mary's complaints. One of the tests that we ordered was a comprehensive stool analysis. Mary had a past history of digestive problems and we also wanted to see if Mary was having a reaction to alpha-gliadin-33-mer, one of the gluten proteins. This test revealed that indeed, Mary was reacting to alpha-gliadin-33-mer. This means every time Mary ingested gluten, her immune system became inflamed, and attacked the gluten like a foreign invader. In Mary's case not only was the body attacking the gluten but also other healthy tissue. We also discovered, after further testing, that Mary had an autoimmune thyroid problem. Mary had a disease called Hashimoto's Thyroiditis, which means her own immune system was attacking her thyroid. One of the main triggers for this autoimmune disease, and all subsequent flare-ups, is gluten. Another scary fact is that those with Hashimoto's are in fact more likely to develop Alzheimer's or other autoimmune diseases, such as Type I diabetes or rheumatoid arthritis.

We began working with Mary and started her on a program. The program consisted of a variety of treatments; one of the initial steps was to eliminate gluten. This was a challenge for Mary since she started each and every day with a bowl of cereal or oatmeal. But she was determined to feel better and improve her health, so she made the change. After the first four weeks of cutting out gluten (in fact, she cut out grains completely) and making a few other changes, Mary lost 24 pounds and her clothes were fitting better. She was so happy and felt like it was easy once she got into the routine and was educated on what to eat.

The results did not end there. Mary felt in increase in her energy level. She was able to make it through her work days and not feel exhausted when she got home. She was also able to enjoy activities with her friends and family that she had missed out on before because of her fatigue. She noticed that her sleep was deep and she was able to stay asleep through the night. This helped her wake up feeling refreshed instead of like she had to drag herself out of bed. Also, just the lightest bump did not create a bruise as it did prior to treatment. Mary was extremely pleased with her results which fueled her motivation to continue with her gluten-free/grain-free lifestyle.

Keeping Kids Happy Around Their Gluten Eating Friends

Children are often the most difficult people to manage when it comes to maintaining a gluten-free diet. This is because they like to go out with their friends, go to pizza parties, go to the movies, and all the while do not want to constantly worry about eating foods that may have gluten. When told they cannot have them at all, they feel completely isolated from their gluten eating friends.

So how can you keep kids happy around their friends, but still maintain a gluten-free lifestyle?

The key is to plan ahead. When your child is going to a birthday party, bring a few gluten-free cupcakes or some gluten-free brownies so he or she can eat a sweet treat with the rest of the kids.

If going out to a pizza restaurant, call ahead and find out if they offer gluten-free options, and order a special pizza just for your child. When the child goes to a friend's house for a sleepover, pack a backpack for him or her that is loaded with gluten-free chips, gluten-free cookies, gluten-free brownies or other fun snacks. This will allow for the full friend experience while still maintaining a safe and healthy lifestyle.

Of course, starting your child out from birth living gluten-free and eating lots of fruits and vegetables helps them to naturally make good choices, even if they are enjoying the occasional dessert or treat.

Remember that although gluten-free treats and grain products are considered 'safe' from the standpoint of gluten, they are not something that should be over-eaten simply because they are gluten-free. These foods are still triggers for diabetes and chronic disease if over-eaten because of the impact they have on blood sugar levels.

Can I Ever Eat Out Again? And, What about Vacations?

DINING OUT

Just as your child may feel a bit out of place or deprived when going out with his or her friends, you too may feel a bit awkward when going out to dinner with a group of friends or colleagues. You may even, after reading about all of the foods that contain gluten, be concerned about how to choose the right foods when dining out in general. Fortunately, this issue is much easier to deal with today than in years past.

The first thing that you should do is check with the restaurant in advance to find out if they offer gluten-free menu options. One way to do this is to check the restaurants website online. More and more local restaurants and even large chains do offer gluten-free options. Many restaurants even have full gluten-free menus. Be sure to be polite, courteous, and friendly with the wait staff. Take your time and clearly explain your dietary needs, and what you would like; most of the time it is no problem at all.

Choose meals that you know all of the ingredients or ask the server to clarify any unknown ingredients. Stay away from dishes with mysterious sauces, salad dressings, and marinades. If ordering dessert, opt for sherbet, sorbet, or a fresh fruit.

Most restaurants will allow you to substitute extra veggies or a salad for a grain. Even if you have to pay an extra couple of dollars, it's worth it in the long run.

Some of the best gluten-free friendly restaurants are the Italian restaurants, despite the fact that they serve pasta, breads and other dough-based foods like pizza. This is because they generally have the healthiest and freshest olive oil that you can pour all over your veggies and salads. They also have great vegetable selections to give you lots of options for your plate.

Essentially, no matter where you eat, you simply design your meal to follow Dr. Steph's Plate Rule©. Many of our patients go to their favorite restaurant and bring with them a small glass bottle that is filled with a home-made dressing. Then, they either order a meal and "redesign" it to have 75% veggies, or they order a salad with some protein on it, and pour their own dressing all over it or just ask for olive oil.

Eating out, while maintaining a gluten-free lifestyle, does not have to be torture. With a little bit of planning and preparation, you will be able to dine with everyone else without a bit of trouble and maintain your health. Check out the list of great restaurants that have gluten-free menus in Appendix A.

VACATIONS

Whenever you're eating a gluten-free diet or suffering with Celiac disease, it can be quite challenging to travel far from home. Special dietary needs have to follow you everywhere, as does Dr. Steph's Plate Rule©, and the only way to go, and enjoy yourself, is to plan ahead.

You can still go on vacation and enjoy great meals and snacks without worrying about what you're eating or about dangerous cross-contamination. All you have to do is prepare yourself for travel so that you can enjoy your vacation and eat well at the same time.

It will take more planning and prepping than simply going out one night to your favorite local restaurant for dinner. This is because you need to consider the length of time that you will be en route to your vacation destination. How long is your flight or drive? When are you going to be where? For example, will you be on a plane during lunch time or when you will need a snack?

The day before your trip, you will want to pack nuts, fruits and dips and veggies for your trip. If you are driving somewhere, you have the luxury of bringing a cooler to keep things fresh. If you are flying, simply pack up your snacks and lunch in disposable containers and, if needed, an ice pack, and you're good to go.

If you are going on a cruise ship, or are staying at a hotel, call ahead to ensure that you can dine on gluten-free foods. Many hotels and cruise lines have many menu items that you can choose from to make eating gluten-free possible while on vacation.

Arm yourself with a list of restaurant chains in the area that you'll be visiting (in the U.S.) so that you know which ones offer gluten-free options. You can go online (before you leave for vacation) and search "gluten-free restaurant chains" and the city that you will be visiting.

Let's say you'll be driving out of state to visit friends or family. You'll want to check out what supermarket chains are in the area you'll be in, so that you know where to shop when you need a few supplies for snacking or making your own meal if you won't be dining out. In general, remember that if you simply follow Dr. Steph's Plate Rule©, you should be fine.

Another great idea is to bring along a supply of gluten-free food bars to use as an emergency meal or snack to keep you eating every 2-3 hours. These are a lifesaver when you're at the airport, or stuck somewhere without access to a decent place to snack or dine. They are great to take with you off the cruise ship while you tour around town.

Some of the most well-known brands for gluten-free snacks are NuGO Free, Kind Bars, Enjoy Life, Bumble Bars and Lara Bars. They can be purchased online or at some retailers. Ener-G Foods produces a great line of single serving gluten-free cereal packages and packets of gluten-free bread (2 slices per pack). We also sell several brands of gluten-free meal replacement bars or meal replacement shake powders, which come in handy if you need to get a meal's worth of nutrients, but are not in a place that has gluten-free foods to eat at that moment. To order these, simply check out our website: MyLivingHealth.com or TheSkinnyDocs.com.

When we travel, which is quite often, we arm ourselves with raw nuts, bars and our whisk/shake cup with a zip-lock baggie of our medical meal replacement shakes (great for breakfast at a hotel that only serves gluten-filled cereal options). This way, in the worst case scenario, we can drink a shake and eat a fruit salad at the hotel (or grab a banana) and we're good to go.

Armed with your list of restaurants that offer great gluten-free items, your supermarket list, snack bars, cereal and bread packets, you'll be more than ready to take a vacation and never have to give a moment's thought worrying about what you're ingesting. Instead, you can sit back and enjoy yourself, bask in the sun, or ski down a powdery hill. You can be secure in the knowledge that you have the "foods and meals" part of the vacation handled and won't have to worry about your nutrition.

RECIPES

Yummy Gluten-Free Snacks

Gluten-Free Kale Chips

1 Large bunch of Kale

4 Tbsp of Macadamia Nut Oil or Olive Oil (just enough to lightly coat each Kale leaf)

Sea Salt

Preheat oven to 300 degrees.

Wash and de-vein the kale leaves. Dry the kale leaves (can be done with a lettuce spinner) and tear into 3-5 inch pieces. In a large bowl add small amount of oil. Pour the kale leaves in the bowl with the oil. Gently toss the leaves, coating them with oil. Lay the kale on baking pans lined with sheets of parchment paper and then lightly sprinkle with sea salt. Bake for 15-20 minutes. Remove and let the cool.

(A note from Dr Tom: These beat out any commercial kale chip. My wife loves them so much she can down an entire head of kale all by herself!)

Gluten-Free Granola Bars

1 1/2 cups Gluten-Free All Purpose Baking Flour

   (see recipe following if you want to make your own)

2 cups Gluten-Free Rolled Oats

1/4 cup Brown Rice Farina

1 cup Apple Juice

2/3 cup Brown Sugar

2/3 cup Applesauce, unsweetened

1/2 tsp Sea Salt

1/2 tsp Cinnamon, ground

1/4 cup Canola Oil, Coconut Oil or Macadamia Nut Oil

1 tsp Gluten-free Vanilla

1/2 cup Pecans

3/4 cup Gluten-Free Chocolate Chips

Butter or Coconut Oil for Pan

Preheat oven to 375 degrees.

Coat a 9 x 13-inch pan with butter or oil. In a large bowl, stir together the flour, oats, farina, cinnamon and salt. Add the brown sugar with a fork. In a separate, smaller bowl stir together the apple juice, applesauce, vanilla, and canola/coconut oil. Add the wet ingredients to the large bowl with the dry ingredients and blend well.

Stir in the nuts and the chocolate chips. Spread the mixture into the oiled pan and flatten with a spoon.

Bake at 375°F for 30 minutes. When done, cut into 24 bars and place on two baking trays, ensuring a bit of space between the bars. Place bars back into the oven and bake an additional 10 minutes. Cool on a wire rack.

Veggies and Hummus

2 cups of Garbanzo Beans

2 cloves Garlic

¼ cup Tahini

Juice of 3 Organic Lemons

1 Tbsp of Parsley, finely chopped

Sea Salt to taste

Add all ingredients to a food processor and blend until smooth.

Slice up some veggies, (red pepper, celery, carrots, broccoli, zucchini, yellow squash, green pepper) and dip in your favorite all natural hummus.

(Make larger batches and freeze for weekly snack rotations)

Fruit Salad

6 ounces Plain or Vanilla Coconut Milk Yogurt (Optional)

1 tsp Chia Seeds

Here is a list of commonly combined fruit, use 4-6 in different combinations

1 cup chopped Apples	½ cup Pineapple
1 cup sliced Bananas	½ cup of Grapes
1/2 cup Blueberries	½ cup of Oranges
1/2 cup chopped Kiwi	Lemon Juice from ½ a lemon, to
1/2 cup sliced Peaches	prevent fruit from turning brown
1/2 cup Strawberries	Shredded Coconut

In a large bowl, mix fruit together. Mix and match the fruit combinations. Add apples, bananas, blueberries, kiwi, peaches, and strawberries and gently add in chia seeds. Serve on top of the coconut yogurt. Garnish with coconut and serve.

Refried Black Bean Dip

2 cups of Organic Black Beans (from canned or from dried)

1 Tbsp Macadamia Nut Oil or Coconut Oil

1 Cooking Onion, chopped

1-2 cloves Garlic

Sea Salt to taste

1-2 Tbsp ground Cumin

In a pot, cook up the chopped onions in the oil on medium-low until cooked/clear. Add the beans, along with about ¼ cup of water. Cook over medium until beans warm. Add the other ingredients and crush the garlic directly into the beans at this point. Cook for a couple minutes, remove from heat, then with a potato masher, mash up the beans until they have the texture of a chunky dip (or go as smooth as you like).

Serve with Taro Chips or Veggies and Guacamole.

Guacamole

2-3 Ripe Organic Avocados

1 small Red Onion, coarsely chopped

Juice of 1 Lime

½ cup Organic Fresh Cilantro, chopped

Sea Salt and Pepper to taste

Place peeled avocados into a mixing bowl. Mash coarsely with a fork or potato masher. Add all the other ingredients and loosely mix. Serve with Taro Chips and Veggie sticks.

Delicious Bean Salad	
1 cup cooked Black Beans	½ Red Pepper, chopped
1 cup cooked Garbanzo Beans	½ Green Pepper, chopped
(or use 2 cups black beans)	½ cup Fresh Cilantro,
1 cup fresh Corn Kernels (from	chopped
frozen ok) – can take out if	1-2 cloves Fresh Garlic,
avoiding grain completely	chopped or crushed
2 whole Carrots, diced	4 Tbsp Olive Oil
2 Celery stalks, diced	2 Tbsp Balsamic Vinegar
1 Red Onion, chopped	Sea Salt and Pepper
Mix all ingredients in a large mixing bowl and serve chilled. 1 cup makes a great snack	

Almond Muffins	
1 cup Butter	2 cups Shredded Coconut
1 cup sliced Raw Almonds	(unsweetened)
1 cup pure Coconut Milk	3 Eggs
(or nut milk)	
Beat and pour in muffin cups. Cook at 400 for 15 minutes.	

Nut Flour Muffins	
1 ¼ cup Nut Flour	1/8 cup Coconut oil
(walnut, almond)	Handful Berries or Shredded
2 Eggs	Fruit (Apple, Peach, etc.)
1 Banana	
Mix all except fruit in food processor and add fruit before pouring into greased muffin tins. Bake at 350 for 12-15 minutes.	

The "Plate Rule" Protein

Meat Loaf Muffins	
1 1/2 lbs Ground Beef or Turkey Breast (I usually triple this recipe and do combos of meats)	3/4 cup of Rice Bread Crumbs or Almond or Walnut Meal, or 1 cup shredded Carrots and Parsley (1/2 cup each)
1 cup Tomato Sauce or Tomato Juice, 1/2 cup of olive tapenade instead or 1 cup finely chopped mixed olives and onions)	1 Egg 1 tsp Dried Basil 1 tsp Dried Oregano 1/2 tsp Pepper
1/2 tsp Sea Salt	

Preheat oven to 350 degrees. In large bowl combine all of above. Form meat mixture on nonstick baking pans into 4 by 2 1/2 by 1 1/4 inch loaves (I'm never exact with this). Bake 30-35 minutes or until centers are 160 degrees (beef) or 170 degrees (turkey). Each loaf makes about 2 servings, so you can eat half at dinner and eat the rest for breakfast or lunch the next day. Serve up with steamed veggies or salad and pour your olive oil dressing over veggies and meat. *Non-stick muffin cups work very well and may not need as much time (20-25 minutes at 375 degrees should work).

**We make up extra-large batches, cook and individually wrap and freeze 2/3 of them to rotate in every other week for meals.

Hoisin Sauce
Heat oil in a large skillet and brown ground chicken/turkey. Add garlic and ginger and saute briefly. Add teriyaki sauce and simmer for 10 minutes while preparing vegetables. Place filling and vegetables in center of a large platter, then surround with lettuce leaves. Serve with Hoisin sauce for dipping. Serves 4.

Gluten-Free Taco Meat

This can be eaten with lettuce or rice wraps or corn shells as tacos, or in rice wraps/paper, or put over a salad of mixed greens, green onions, chopped red peppers, and topped with crushed Taro Chips (for crunch).

2 lbs ground Turkey, Chicken, Lamb or grass-fed Beef

Cook up the meat in a pan until cooked through.

In a mixing cup, mix together the following spices and herbs (assuming all are organic):

2 Tbsp ground Chili Powder	½ tsp Garlic Powder
1 Tbsp ground Cumin	½ tsp Onion Powder
½ tsp Sea Salt	1 Tbsp Tapioca Starch (a Gluten-Free Thickener)

Add 3/4 cup water and mix well. Set ground meat to low, and pour in the seasoning mixture. Stir until thickened (a few minutes). Serve as suggested above.

Asian Chicken Lettuce Wraps

1 tablespoon olive

1 pound ground chicken or can also try ground turkey

2 tablespoons crushed garlic

2 tablespoons finely shredded ginger

2/3 cup Teriyaki Sauce

Vegetables for filling: grated carrots, mung bean sprouts, sliced Radish, julienned cucumber

Boston or romaine lettuce leaves, rinsed and dried

Spaghetti Sauce 'Chili'

What I discovered is that food is all about the sauce. This is especially true for Spaghetti Sauce. It's not the filler flavorless gluten-filled noodles that I craved, but the yummy sauce. So, I started making it extra chunky, like a chili, and eating it that way with side salad or lots of steamed veggies. Some even go so far as to bake up a Spaghetti Squash to replace the noodles. If you really want noodles, I would recommend Buckwheat Pasta (100%). Buckwheat is gluten-free, and the pasta is very tasty and very filling.

If Tomatoes are not on your list, then cook up the ground meat, add the veggies and spices/herbs and serve without the tomatoes. No big deal...the oregano, onions and garlic season the meat nicely. You can even add chopped red and green peppers and mushrooms.

2 lbs ground Grass-Fed Beef (or 1 lbs each of Beef and Buffalo)	1-2 Tbsp Organic Dried Oregano Crushed (I like a LOT of oregano, but add to taste.)
1 whole Onion chopped	
1 cup chopped Green Pepper	1 Tbsp Organic Dried Basil Crushed
2-4 cloves Garlic (I like my sauce really garlicky)	1 tsp Organic Dried Thyme Crushed
1 can Organic diced Tomatoes (large)	
	1-2 Bay Leaves
1 can Organic Tomato Sauce (could even be a jar of organic marinara sauce)	1-2 tsp Sea Salt (to taste)

*A note from Dr. Steph: Here's where you make stuff up and add as much or little tomato sauce and canned tomatoes depending on how 'thick' and chunky you like it. I like mine really meaty and thick, so I don't use a ton of tomatoes.

Cook the meat, onions, green pepper (mushrooms) until meat is brown (I add garlic after meat is cooked when I'm adding everything else). Drain the fat. Stir in everything else. Garlic should be fresh crushed/pressed right into the sauce. Reduce heat and simmer for maybe 15-20 minutes. Because I use less tomato/liquid, it won't need to simmer as long. Serve on a plate or in a bowl with your steamed veggies. No need for pasta, since the sauce is thick and meaty enough to stand alone. IF you want pasta that is also not going to add calories or spike your sugars, you can serve this with Miracle Noodles (found at most health food stores or online), which are made from the starch of a root vegetable but contains almost no sugar/carbs/calories at all!

Don't forget to pick out that bay leaf!

Bison and Bean Chili

1/2 pound ground bison	2 teaspoons ground cumin
1 large onion, finely chopped	2 tablespoons chili powder
1 large carrot, finely chopped	1 tablespoon apple cider vinegar
1/2 small head cauliflower, stemmed and cut into small florets (about 3 cups)	1 (15-ounce) can no-salt-added diced tomatoes
1 medium green bell pepper, stemmed, seeded and finely chopped	1 (28-ounce) can no-salt-added crushed tomatoes
3 large garlic cloves, finely chopped	1 (15-ounce) can no-salt-added kidney beans, drained and rinsed
	1/2 cup loosely packed cilantro leaves, chopped

Heat a large Dutch oven or pot over high heat. When the pot is very hot, add bison and brown it, stirring often for 5 minutes. Add onion and carrot, and cook, until both begin to soften, about 5 minutes. Add 1/2 cup water to deglaze the pan, scraping brown bits from the bottom of the pan as the water evaporates.

Add cauliflower, bell pepper and garlic and cook until vegetables begin to soften, about 5 minutes. Add cumin, chili powder, vinegar, tomatoes and beans along with 1 cup water. Bring to a boil, then reduce to a simmer and cover, stirring occasionally, until vegetables are fork tender, about 45 minutes.

Serve garnished with chopped cilantro. Serves 4-6.

Baked Chicken with Spinach and Pears

4 boneless, skinless chicken breasts	4 to 6 cups (1 large bunch) loosely packed spinach (not baby), washed, dried, stems removed
Sea salt and freshly ground black pepper	
3 tablespoons extra-virgin olive oil, divided	2 tablespoons apple cider vinegar
1/2 cup diced red onion	2 ripe Anjou pears, peeled, cored and cut into 1/2-inch-thick slices
2 tablespoons chopped fresh parsley	

Preheat oven to 375°F. Generously season each chicken breast with salt and pepper. In a large, oven-proof skillet heat 1 tablespoon olive oil and sear breasts 2 to 3 minutes each side until lightly golden. Place pan in oven and bake until chicken is cooked through, about 15 minutes.

While chicken is cooking, heat 1 tablespoon olive oil in a large pan over medium heat and sauté red onion until just softened, 2 to 3 minutes. Add spinach and toss until wilted. Season with salt and pepper and transfer to a large platter or divide evenly between 4 plates. Wipe out pan and heat remaining 1 tablespoon olive oil with vinegar. Add pears and gently heat until warm. Stir in parsley. Arrange cooked chicken breasts on spinach. Top with warmed pear slices. 4 Servings.

Gluten-Free Fish Ideas

- Organic Salmon Marinade from Vital Choice/vitalchoice.com (good on any fish)
- Ground Macadamia Nuts with 1 slice cooked Turkey Bacon (pack on fish and bake)
- Marinade fish for 30 minutes in a warmed mixture of melted butter, olive oil, fresh lemon juice or dry white wine, chopped onion, crushed garlic and freshly chopped dill.
- Spread a GF Indian sauce or tomato or artichoke bruschetta over the fish and bake as usual. These can be found at stores like Whole Foods or Trader Joe's.

Generally, most fresh fish can be baked at 425 degrees for 10-13 minutes depending on how cooked you like your fish, and whether you have a lot of sauce on it or not. It depends on your oven.

Marinades for chicken, fish or whatever

Citrus Marinade	
½ cup each fresh Lemon and Lime Juice	2 tsp ground Pepper
	2 crushed Bay Leaves
¼ cup Macadamia Nut or Avocado Oil	3 Tbsp chopped Cilantro
	4 cloves Garlic, crushed
Mix all in shallow wide mixing bowl. Add food and marinate 1-2 hours (less for fish, more for chicken). Bake or grill as desired. Modified from a recipe by Joel Schwartz	

Coconut Marinade	
1/3 cup Coconut Milk	1 tsp Stevia
2 Tbsp Lime Juice	2 Tbsp Fresh Ginger Root, finely grated
Combine all and marinate steak, chicken, shrimp or fish. Barbeque and baste with sauce throughout.	

Mojo Criollo	
1/3 cup Macadamia Nut Oil	½ tsp ground Cumin
6-8 cloves Garlic minced/crushed	¼ tsp Lime Rind
2/3 cup Lime Juice	Salt and Pepper to taste
Combine all and marinate choice of meat.	
Modified From "Miami Spice" cookbook	

Tandoori Marinade	
½ cup Coconut Milk 2 Tbsp each Lemon and Lime Juice 2 tsp Sea Salt 2 cloves Garlic, minced/ crushed 1 tsp Ginger minced/grated	½ tsp each Cumin, Coriander Seed, Cayenne Pepper ¼ tsp each Turmeric, Black Pepper 1/8 tsp Cinnamon Pinch ground Cloves
Mix all making sure well blended. Marinade meat of choice for several hours. Use leftover sauce for basting while grilling/cooking.	

Beef Teriyaki Marinade	
Scale this recipe as you need to for however much meat you are marinating. Beef tenderloin is the best in our opinion and grills up nicely.	
1 cup Wheat-/Gluten-Free Soy Sauce 2 cups Water ½ cup (to taste) Blackstrap Molasses	2-4 Tbsp Fresh Ginger, grated (keep a root in freezer and grate as needed) 1 Tbsp Dried Mustard
Combine all and marinate.	

To change up the above recipes/marinade, simply use different fresh herbs: dill, tarragon, parsley, cilantro, etc.

Soy-free, Gluten-Free Stir Fry Sauce

1 cup of Wheat-/Gluten-Free Chicken Broth 2 -3 Tbsp of Almond Butter or Cashew Butter 1 Tbsp Tapioca Starch, Corn Starch or Arrowroot (to thicken)	1-2 Tbsp (I mostly guess) Toasted Sesame Oil 1-2 cloves Garlic, crushed 1 Tbsp grated Fresh Organic Ginger (keep a root in freezer and grate as needed)

Mix above ingredients together in a measuring cup. Stir fry up your meat with macadamia nut oil, then put meat aside into a bowl. Return stir fry pan to stove top and add more oil to stir fry up the veggies.

Add the meat once veggies are almost done, then reduce heat to medium or med/low and add sauce. Cover and simmer until thickened.

Serve as is or with ½ cup of brown rice or rice noodles.

Remember the Plate Rule when making stir fry: ¾ veggies, ¼ meat.

Gluten-Free Soy Stir Fry Sauce #2

½ cup Wheat-/Gluten-Free Soy Sauce ½ cup Water or Broth 2 Tbsp Toasted Sesame Oil	1-2 Tbsp Fresh grated Ginger (optional) 1-2 cloves Fresh crushed Garlic (optional) 1 Tbsp Tapioca Starch

Mix above ingredients together in a measuring cup. Stir fry your meat with macadamia nut oil, then put meat aside into a bowl. Return stir fry pan to stove top and add more oil to stir fry the veggies.

Add the meat once veggies are almost done, then reduce heat to medium or med/low and add sauce. Cover and simmer until thickened. Serve as is or with ½ cup of brown rice or rice noodles.

Remember Dr. Steph's Plate Rule© when making stir fry: ¾ veggies, ¼ meat.

The Veggies Meal Plate

The easiest way to do veggies, which is often our default method during busy weekdays, is to simply steam your veggies and serve them with the Olive Oil Dressing (The basic recipe and a variation are on page 103) drizzled all over them. Great vegetables for steaming include: Broccoli, asparagus, kale, chard, spinach, beet greens. Always keep a large batch of dressing on hand and ready to pour over steamed veggies or salad.

Others veggies seem to be better lightly sautéed in butter, macadamia nut oil or coconut oil. Add mushrooms, peppers, onions, garlic, zucchini, asparagus, etc. however you like it!

No recipe needed for many of these, but here are some yummy ones for salads:

Caesar Salad
In a large wooden salad bowl (that you will use for serving) mix:

Yolk of one Egg (the white can be cooked and tossed in later or whatever) 1 Fresh crushed Garlic clove (or 2 if you like really garlicky) 1 Tbsp Dijon Mustard (try to get gluten-free)	2 tsp Gluten-Free Fish Sauce (whole foods) or Anchovy Paste Juice of one small Lemon or 1/2 large one (depends on how tangy you want it)

Whisk everything together in the bowl until it's like a thick sauce. Slowly pour in olive oil while whisking until you have it to taste (here's where you can adjust for lemon tanginess) - about 1/2 cup to 3/4 cup)

Once done, you can now pour into the dressing about 1/2 cup fresh grated parmesan. Toss into the bowl three chopped up 'heads' of organic romaine lettuce and toss until the lettuce is well covered/mixed with the dressing.

If you need to be gluten –free but want croutons, then use rice bread or other gluten-free bread for croutons, or none at all. Taro chips sprinkled on top will add crunch with no worries about gluten.

This is great with rotisserie or grilled chicken or grass-fed beef tenderloin. I like the chicken right on the salad....when in a hurry, get a roaster chicken from Whole Foods and just tear up the chicken onto the salad - yum!

Roasted Vegetables
A variety of vegetables can be used in this recipe, just cut them to a similar size. Suggested vegetables are butternut squash, sweet potatoes, eggplant, onions, carrots, asparagus, beets, etc.
Preheat oven to 400 degrees. Place the large chunks of veggies on a baking sheet. Coat with olive or macadamia nut oil, salt and pepper and bake until veggies are tender. These are good at room temperature as well as hot. You can also do these on the grill. Also nice with crushed fresh garlic added to the oil before coating.

Yummy Mixed Greens Salad	
Prewashed organic mixed greens (amount depends on how many people you're serving. 1 small box to 1 large box should do it	
1 cup thinly sliced fresh organic basil leaves (or more if you like) 1-2 roasted red peppers (peeled) - either roast on grill or in oven until skin burned/crisp, then peel the skin off) - sliced thinly (can also buy in jars)	1 small herbed goat cheese crumbled on top of salad (optional if dairy intolerant) 5 green onions chopped (or more if you like onions) Balsamic dressing (1/2 cup olive oil, 2 tbsp. balsamic vinegar, 2 cloves fresh crushed garlic, pinch of sea salt)
Toss it up...	

The "Plate Rule" Starches

I'm of the mindset—and of the reality that many of us have limited time to cook—to keep things very simple. You can use easy and uncomplicated recipes for starchy veggies: simply bake sweet potatoes and keep them on hand in the fridge to re-heat as needed, steamed or raw carrots, sliced avocado either in your salad, or right onto the plate as your side veggie, etc. Remember to limit this on your Plate to 0-1/2 cup to avoid elevating your blood sugar too much.

The following are some great recipes for when you have time.

Butternut Squash Soup	
1 whole large Butternut Squash, peeled and cubed, or about 6-8 cups of already peeled and cubed butternut squash from the grocery store	Enough Gluten-Free Chicken Broth to cover the squash in the pot (about 8-10 cups depending on how thick you like your soup)
1 large Onion chopped	1 tsp Sea Salt
2 Tbsp Macadamia Nut or Coconut Oil	Ground Nutmeg to garnish

In a large soup pot, cook the onions on low in the oil until they are soft (5-10 minutes), but not burnt. Add the squash and cover the squash with the broth. Add the salt, cover and bring to a boil, reduce heat, stir and simmer on low for about 40 minutes. With a hand-mixer, blend the softened squash until your soup is silky-smooth. Serve and garnish with ground nutmeg. Remember, as per Plate Rule, that ½ cup will be a serving since the squash is a starch that can spike blood sugars if too much is consumed.

Beet Salad	
6 Organic Beets	1-2 crushed cloves Garlic
Olive Oil	½ cup chopped Fresh Dill
Juice of 1 Lemon	Sea Salt and Pepper to taste
Wash/scrub the beets clean (cut off tips) and boil in a large pot of water until cooked through (about 15 minutes depending on size of beets (fork test them). Peel and cube beets into 1 inch cubes and put into large mixing bowl. Toss with enough Olive Oil to coat well, then add the lemon juice, salt and pepper, garlic and dill and mix well. Serve warm or leftover cold as a ½ cup side dish.	

Turnip Slaw	
2 Turnips, shredded	1 Tbsp Lemon Juice
2 Tbsp Olive Oil	Sea Salt and Pepper to taste
Toss all above ingredients and serve with meal	

Sweet Potato Apple Bake

This one is a big hit for holiday dinners.

Bake sweet potatoes wrapped in foil on 400 degrees for about an hour (depending on size - bake until soft to touch). I usually do 4 or 5 for a large crock pot (mine is a big oval thing)

Peel about 6 apples (but buy more, b/c you can always peel more if you need more to balance) - I like Macintosh or something else a little on the tart side)

Once potatoes are baked, peel and slice into 1 to 1 ½ inch thick 'medallion's and layer on the bottom of the crock pot.

Then, place large slices / chunks of the peeled apples on top of layer of potatoes to make a second layer

Cut small chunks of butter over the apples, sprinkle some cinnamon and nutmeg and a little stevia sprinkled on layer (not a lot - this stuff is super sweet)

keep repeating the layers this way until crock pot is full

put on low - let it warm down until apples are soft and cooked (usually a couple of hours)

serve right out of the crock pot

Salad Dressings

A Basic Olive Oil Dressing
3 parts Olive Oil
2 parts Lemon Juice
1-2 tsp Gluten-Free Dijon Mustard
Salt, Pepper to taste
1 clove Garlic, minced
(may add dash of stevia for 'honey mustard')
Add ingredients to a jar and shake well. Refrigerate for up to 1 week. Use for salads, for meat salads (chicken, tuna, etc.), and pour on steamed veggies. Ideally, you should steam veggies on rotation for each dinner and this dressing is great for pouring on them. You can also keep out the mustard and add dried green herbs to change up, or use lime juice instead of lemon juice for a change of taste.

Olive Oil Dressing Variation This gluten-free dressing is one that you can make up for salads or to pour over steamed, baked or grilled veggies:
1 cup Organic, Extra Virgin, Cold Pressed Olive Oil
1-2 cloves Garlic, crushed
1-2 tsp Green Herbs (mixtures of tarragon, oregano, basil, etc)
¼ tsp Sea Salt (or to taste)
Make this mixture up in a glass jar or bottle and leave in cupboard to easily and liberally pour onto your veggies and salad every day. You can add fresh squeezed lemon, lime or grapefruit juice or a splash of balsamic or cider vinegar to jazz it up. Don't add these to the entire dressing unless you are going to refrigerate the dressing. I like leaving the oil mixture out because the oil hardens in the fridge, making me less likely to use it and to eat my veggies (they taste so much better with the dressing). Experiment with different herbs and juice/vinegar combos.

Gluten-Free Dessert Recipes

Gluten-Free Flour
Equal amounts of soy and tapioca flour plus twice that amount of brown rice flour. Add 1 teaspoon of a "gluten substitute" such as guar gum, xanthum gum or "Pre-gel" starch. These can be obtained at most health food stores.

Another flour mix to try is:	
2 cups Sorghum Flour	1/2 cup Sweet Rice Flour
2 cups Brown Rice Flour (I use superfine brown rice flour)	1/2 cup Tapioca Flour
	1/2 cup Amaranth Flour
1 1/2 cups Potato Starch, not Potato Flour	1/2 cup Quinoa Flour
1/2 cup White Rice Flour	

Banana "Ice-Cream"
2 Bananas, sliced and frozen
1 cup unsweetened Vanilla Almond Milk
2 Tbsp Smooth Almond Butter
Put bananas, almond milk and almond butter into a blender or use a hand mixer. Purée, turning off the motor and stirring the mixture two or three times, until it is smooth and creamy. Pour into two bowls and serve.

Chocolate Chia Seed Pudding
2/3 cup whole Chia Seeds
2 cups Chocolate Coconut Milk
In a glass bowl add the chia seeds and coconut milk. Mix together with a fork. Place top on the bowl and place in the refrigerator overnight. The next day mix together with a fork and serve.

Flourless Brownies Makes 32 (this is a double batch)	
2 (15-ounce) can no-salt-added Black Beans, drained and rinsed 6 large Eggs 1 cup Organic Coconut Oil, more for the baking dish (melted) 1/2 cup Raw Organic Cocoa Powder 1/4 tsp non-iodized Sea Salt 4 tsp Wheat-/Gluten-Free Vanilla Extract	1 cup Cane Sugar or Raw Brown Sugar or 2-4 Tbsp Stevia (see conversion charts online) 1 cup Wheat-/Gluten-Free Semi-Sweet Chocolate Chips 2/3 cup finely chopped Walnuts (or, if issue with nuts, another cup of chocolate chips)

Preheat oven to 350°F.

Butter a 12x9-inch baking pan. Place the black beans, eggs, melted oil, cocoa powder, salt, vanilla extract and sugar in the bowl of a food processor and blend until smooth. Remove the blade and gently stir in the chocolate chips and walnuts. Transfer mixture to the prepared pan. Bake the brownies for 35-40 minutes, or until just set in the center. Cool before cutting into squares.

Gluten-Free Chocolate Cake

5 large Eggs

8 oz Unsweetened Chocolate

4 oz Semisweet Chocolate

1 1/3 cups Sugar, divided

1 cup Butter or Coconut Oil

1/2 cup Water

Preheat oven to 350 o. Lightly coat a 9-inch spring form pan with butter. Crack the eggs into a small glass or metal bowl and temper them over low heat on the stove, but do not cook. This will allow the eggs to triple in volume when beaten.

In a medium pan, melt the chocolate, water, 1 cup sugar, and butter over medium heat, stirring continually. Remove from heat and let cool. Transfer the eggs to a mixing bowl. Add the remaining 1/3 cup sugar to the eggs and beat until tripled in volume. Fold the chocolate mixture. Pour the mixture into the prepared pan and bake 30-35 minutes; it will be a little loose in center. Serve warm or room temperature.

Carrot Cake

6 Eggs, separated

½ cup Honey or Grade B Maple Syrup

1 ½ cup Cooked and Pureed Carrot

1 Tbsp Grated Orange Rind

1 Tbsp Fresh Lemon Juice

3 cups Almond Flour

Preheat oven to 325o. Beat egg yolks and honey/syrup together. Mix in carrot puree, orange rind and lemon juice and almond flour. Beat the egg whites until stiff and fold into cake batter. Spoon into greased loose bottom 9 inch springform pan and bake for 50 minutes or until fork tests clean. Cool in pan 15 mins, then turn out onto wire rack to cool completely.

Almond Pecan Pie Crust*
1 cup Almonds   ½ cup Pecans   1/3 cup Pitted Soft Dates   3 Tbsp Water

In separate bowls, cover almonds and pecans with water and soak for 8-12 hours (overnight). Drain and rinse. In a food processor, grind almonds to consistency of moist meal. Place in a medium-size bowl and set aside. Do the same to the pecans, then mix into the almonds. In the processor blend dates and water until smooth, then stir into nut mixture thoroughly mixed and dough-like. Shape into a ball and place on 12" length of wax paper. Top with another 12" piece of wax paper. Flatten ball with hand, then using rolling pin, roll out dough into an 11" circle. Carefully remove the top paper, invert into an oiled 9" pie plate, pressing gently. Trim excess crust and press gently to even the edges. Place crust in a food dehydrator set at 125 o for 2 hours (or preheat oven to 250 o, then turn off and let crust sit in oven with door closed until dry and set (about 30 minutes)). It will still be sticky and very moist and will fall apart when cut, but who cares because it tastes good.

*Recipe from Spring 1994 Vegetarian Gourmet – from the Green City Market & Café in Washington, DC; chef Aris LaTham.

Gluten-Free Breakfast

Your gluten-free breakfast should follow the Dr. Steph's Plate Rule©. As we mentioned earlier, having left overs from dinner for breakfast is a great way to start the day. This is difficult, at first, for many of our patients. But once they get their body used to it they could not image going back to that bowl of cereal or oatmeal.

If you prefer "breakfast" type items you can choose from GF turkey bacon, chicken or turkey sausage, grass-fed beef bacon. Scrambled or boiled eggs are also a good source of protein in the morning. Also make sure you include some veggies. These may include sautéed spinach and onions, steamed broccoli or steamed kale.

Breakfast Smoothie	
1 Serving of Pea or Rice or Denatured Whey Protein Powder 1 Serving of "Green" Powder ½ of a banana 1 Tbsp of Raw Unsalted Almond Butter	¼ cup of frozen berries (blueberries, raspberries etc.) 1 Tbsp of ground flax seed 6 oz of filtered water 4 oz of unsweetened almond milk
Use a hand mixer or blender to blend. This is a quick and easy breakfast option. Be creative and mix up the ingredients in your breakfast smoothie. Other ingredients may include coconut milk, coconut butter, hemp protein powder, cherries, lemon or lime juice and chia seeds. If you are feeling a bit adventurous you can add a couple Swiss chard or kale leaves.	

We are including a couple of pancake recipes but these should not be eaten on a daily or weekly basis. These should be eaten on rare occasions and always include the other parts of the plate rule.

Gluten/Grain Free Pancakes
1 Egg ¼ cup ground Almonds ¼ cup Coconut Milk
Combine and cook as regular pancakes in coconut butter or grass fed cow butter (if ok with dairy)

Blueberry Walnut Pancakes	
½ cup finely ground Walnuts (like course flour) Sea Salt ½ tsp Baking Powder (aluminum free from whole foods or health food store)	1 Egg ½ cup Filtered Water 1 ½ tsp Macadamia Nut Oil Chopped Walnuts and Organic Blueberries
Make so batter is thick enough to 'support' the fruit and nut. Cook in a little butter or macadamia nut oil, flip once and serve with grade "B" maple syrup.	

7-Day Gluten-Free Sample Menu

The following is a sample seven day gluten-free menu. It is assumed that all of the ingredients used are gluten-free. There are no absolutes to using this menu, so you can mix and match lunches and dinners, or make creative changes as necessary. After you get accustomed to this type of schedule, start putting in other gluten-free recipes that you, and your family, enjoy. The trick is to rotate foods around and to not get stuck eating the same foods every day.

Also keep in mind that depending on your schedule you may also need a snack in the morning between breakfast and lunch. Ideally you do not want to go without eating more than 3 hours. This will help you keep your blood sugar stable, help reduce fatigue and cravings, and prevent diabetes. This menu is designed to give you something easy to follow and something to get started with.

Day 1	
Breakfast:	Two eggs with sautéed zucchini, mushroom and onions
Snack	10 raw walnuts and ½ cup-1 cup of fresh organic blueberries
Lunch	Turkey sandwich on gluten-free bread (or leaves of lettuce if going completely grain-free) with, avocado and roasted red peppers, lettuce and a side of sweet potato chips
Snack	Veggies and Hummus
Dinner	Salmon Filet, steamed broccoli, and spinach with olive oil dressing

Day 2	
Breakfast:	Cream of Buckwheat with berries/fruit
Snack	Sliced Apple with Almond butter
Lunch	Grilled Chicken Breast on a Salad
Snack	Veggie sticks and ½ cup black bean dip
Dinner	Beef Taco Meat on a salad of lettuce, tomatoes, avocado, with crumbled Taro Chips on top

Day 3	
Breakfast:	Pea/Rice/Whey Protein Shake blended with Almond butter and frozen organic berries and veggie/green powder
Snack	Pear
Lunch	Ground beef with onions, lettuce, tomatoes (left over from night before)
Snack	Couple tablespoons pumpkin seeds
Dinner	Baked Cod with sautéed onions, green zucchini, yellow squash and ½ cup baked sweet potato

Day 4	
Breakfast:	2 Scrambled eggs with steamed spinach
Snack	Fruit Salad
Lunch	Gluten-free fish sticks, baby carrots and broccoli with hummus
Snack	Gluten-free granola/snack bar
Dinner	Halibut filet with rice, sautéed or steamed kale with garlic olive oil dressing

Day 5	
Breakfast:	GF Turkey Sausage with steamed Asparagus
Snack	10 Organic Cherries and ¼ cup Raw Cashews
Lunch	Roasted Chicken sliced on gluten-free bread (or leaf lettuce if going grain-free) with hummus spread.
Snack	Taro chips with guacamole
Dinner	T-Bone steak (grass-fed), ½ cup beet salad, steamed broccoli with olive oil dressing

Day 6	
Breakfast:	GF Chicken sausage with red/green peppers
Snack	Plain or Vanilla coconut yogurt with berries
Lunch	2 Boiled eggs chopped over salad
Snack	Kale chips and nectarine
Dinner	Salmon, steamed Brussels sprouts and beet salad

Day 7	
Breakfast:	2 egg omelet with turkey bacon, onions, mushrooms
Snack	2 Plums or Fresh Figs
Lunch	1 slice (or half a mini) Meat loaf with a small salad
Snack	GF Granola Bar
Dinner	Grilled chicken breast with sautéed Swiss Chard or Beet Greens in onions and ½ cup butternut squash soup

Conclusion

We are passionate about helping people improve their health, prevent chronic disease, and reduce, and eliminate, the need for medications, through natural means. There is a time and a place for the use of medications, but the majority of the prescribed medications, we believe, can be reduced and eliminated, with the appropriate intervention and treatment. When the body is given the right environment and the correct tools it can heal itself. But when your body is neglected for months, or years, it can be difficult to know what the body needs to be healthy. There is so much health information out there that sometimes it is confusing and frustrating. We have seen, time and again in our practice, clinical results using the information and tools provided here. We believe these same tools and information will also help you.

The information provided here shows just how easy it is to go gluten-free. The gluten-free lifestyle offers many health benefits beyond having fewer digestive issues. Rhere are a number of reasons to cut gluten out of your diet. From lowering your risk for many debilitating diseases, to having healthier children.

Since more and more people are seeking knowledge and are going gluten-free and grain-free, the food choices have gotten more plentiful, restaurants have come on board, and meals are quite delicious.

Now is the time to take action. You cannot keep doing the same things and eating the same food, if you want different results. You must start making changes, if you want to see different outcomes. If you have not already started making changes, then start today.

The research on this subject continues to be published and is continually evolving. We are dedicated to keeping up on the latest research to help us provide the best care possible for our patients and for ourselves. It is important that you dedicate yourself to improving your own health by expanding your knowledge. Remember, you are responsible for your health. If you put that responsibility in someone else's hands, like the health insurance company or the pharmaceutical companies, it is you, not them, who must live with the results. Educate yourself, ask questions, take an active role in getting healthy and keep persisting until you are happy with your outcome.

Be patient. Rome wasn't built in a day. Being and staying healthy is a continual process. In time, you will realize this lifestyle change is quite simple and takes just a bit of extra planning, but the difference you will feel in your own body will astound you!

APPENDIX A:
Gluten-Free Restaurants

** You still need to watch the dressings, seasonings and sauces as many restaurants qualify as Gluten-free (GF) simply by not having wheat or other similar grains on the plate and not accounting for MSG. The list of restaurants that are providing gluten-free menus or options is growing by the day, so when in doubt, simply ask the server if the restaurant has a gluten-free menu. If not, simply follow the Plate Rule and make modifications to the menu as needed.

Also remember to ask your local liquor store for gluten-free beer options, or simply switch to drinking organic, sulfate-free red wine, which at least contains heart healthy antioxidants and so is better for you than beer anyway.

Austin Grill	Legal Sea Foods
Bertucci's	Not Your Average Joe's
Biaggi's	On the Border
Bonefish Grill	Outback Steakhouse
BJ's Restaurant & Brewhouse	P.F. Chang's China Bistro
Boston Market	Picazzo's
Carrabbas	Pizza Fusion
Cheeseburger in Paradise	Rockfish Seafood Grill
(also has grass-fed beef burgers)	Ruby Tuesday
Chick-Fil-A	Sam & Louie's
Chili's	Ted's Montana Grill
Fresh To Order	Uno Chicago Grill
Garlic Jim's	Wildfire
Glory Days Grill	Z'Tejas Southwestern Grill
Gordon Biersch	

Appendix B:
Gluten-Free Grocery Shopping

It is very easy to do an internet search for grocery stores and food markets that offer gluten-free choices. Here are some examples in our area:

- David's Natural Market
- Giant
- Publix
- Safeway
- Sprouts
- Sunflower
- The Fresh Market
- Trader Joe's
- Wegman's
- Whole Foods
- Wild Oats

Online shopping is something we do a lot for health and convenience. Here's a limited list of places to get GF and healthy food options:

- **vitalchoice.com** (where we get our wild Alaskan fish and seafood and GF herb marinade)
- **uswellnessmeats.com** (where we get our grass-fed/finished meats and poultry, as well as unpasteurized cheeses from grass-fed cows)

Appendix C:
Gluten-Free on the outside

It's important to remember that your skin and hair products should also be GF. Look for the same ingredients that you would rule out when looking for packaged foods, such as hydrolyzed wheat, wheat protein, etc. Here are some of Dr. Steph's favorites, along with a limited list of other options:

- **afterglowcosmetics.com** for make-up
- **keyssoap.com** for sunblock, shampoo, skin lotion
- Remember that plain old coconut oil is a great shaving cream and skin lotion – even for the face.

Appendix D:
Gluten-Free Food Category Lists

Here's a list of examples (not a complete list, but enough to help you determine what foods go where) of foods and how to categorize them to easily follow Dr. Steph's Plate Rule©.

Remember to follow Dr. Steph's Plate Rule© for choosing where to put these foods. The top 3 categories (meats and veggies) generally go on your Meal Plates (along with the oils), while the Beans, Fruits and Nuts or combos of these foods generally get eaten for snacks.

Meal Plate Foods:

CONCENTRATED PROTEIN

Average size 3-6 oz.

1 serving = 150 calories

Servings per day: 3-6

Cooked or as indicated (grilled, baked, roasted, poached, sautéed, stir-fried).

All fish should be wild, poultry free-range and red meat grass-fed when possible.

- Beef, Lamb, Venison, Buffalo/Bison, Veal, Goat
- Salmon, Cod, Halibut, Rainbow Trout, Red Snapper, Sardines, Swordfish, Whitefish, White and Yellow Perch, Yellowtail, Albacore (Tuna), Anchovy, Flounder, Grouper, Haddock, Mahimahi, Pickerel, Sea Bass, Sea Trout
- Scallops, Crab, Lobster, Shrimp, etc.
- Chicken, Turkey, Cornish Hen, Duck, Quail
- Eggs (2-4 per week)

STICKS AND LEAVES VEGGIES

Average Serving Size = 1/2 cup or more

10-25 calories

Servings per Day—Unlimited or 50-75% of the Meal Plate

Artichoke, Arugula, Asparagus, Broccoli, Brussel Sprouts, Cabbage, Celery, Cucumber, Fiddlehead Ferns, Ginger, Greens (collards, kale, chards, beet or turnip greens, spinach, dandelion, parsley), Fennel, Lettuces, Mushrooms, Okra, Onions, Peppers, Radicchio, Radishes, All Sprouts, Tomato, Watercress, Zucchini, Green Olives

**Beans and corn are not veggies. Corn is a grain (gluten-free) and beans are legumes.

STARCHY VEGGIES

Average Serving Size = 1/2 cup and

Approx 45 calories

Servings—1-2 per day

- Sweet Potato
- Pumpkin
- Turnips
- Avocado
- Beets
- Carrots
- Yams
- All other squashes

**White potato is not on the list because this is one of the worst culprits for spiking blood sugar.

OILS

Average Serving Size = 1 Teaspoon

Approximately 40 calories

Servings—4-7 per day

All oils should be organic, cold-pressed, extra-virgin.

You can cook with the following oils:

- Sesame Oil
- Macadamia Nut Oil
- Grapeseed Oil

- Coconut Oil

Don't cook with these oils—use them as dressings instead:

- Olive Oil
- Flax Oil
- Fish Oil

THE SNACK FOODS

FRUITS

1 Serving Approximately 80 calories

Servings—1-2 per day

- Fresh or Frozen Organic Apple, 1 medium
- Apricot, 3 med
- Berries: 1 cup blueberries, raspberries or blackberries
- Banana (1/2 large or 1 small)
- Cherries, 10
- Figs (2)
- Grapefruit, 1 whole
- Grapes, 15
- Mango, 1/2 med
- Orange (1 large, 2 small)
- Peaches, 2 small
- Pear, 1 med
- Pineapple (1/2 cup)
- Plum (2 small)
- Watermelon (2 cups)
- Lemons/Limes

NUTS AND SEEDS

Approximately 100 calories

Servings—1-2 per day

- Walnuts, 7-8
- Pumpkin seeds, 2 Tbs

- Almond, Pecan, Hazelnut: 10-12
- Macadamia, 7-8
- Sesame, Pine nut, Peanuts, Pistachio 2 Tbsp
- Nut butters (peanut, almond, etc): 1 Tbsp

BEANS AND LEGUMES

Ideally from dried and soaked 24-48 hrs.

Average serving size = 1/2 cup

1 serving = 110 calories

Serving Size: 0-1 per day

- Adzuki beans, Pinto Beans, Black-Eyed Peas
- Black Beans, Broad Beans, Fava Beans, Garbanzo Beans, Green Beans, Lima Beans, Northern Beans, Red Beans, String Beans, White Beans, Green Peas, Pea Pods

GRAINS/BREADS

Average Serving Size = 1/2 cup cooked

Approximately 75-100 calories

Servings—0-1 per day

- Rice or other (1/4-1/2 cup cooked)
- Rice cake (1)
- Rice wrap (gluten-free) (1)
- Rice crackers (5-10)
- Gluten-Free flours

Other gluten-free grains: buckwheat, amaranth, quinoa, millet, gluten-free oat

DAIRY

Average Serving Size 2oz or 1/2 cup shredded

Approximately 80-150 calories

Servings—0-1 per day

Choose unpasteurized dairy products from grass-fed cows or goats i.e. cheese, yogurts, butter, cream, milk.

OTHER FOODS

CONDIMENTS/SPICES/HERBS

Cayenne, Curry, Dulse, Kelp, Turmeric, Carob, Allspice, Anise, Arrowroot, Basil, Bay Leaf, Cardamom, Carob, Cayenne, Chives, Chocolate/Cacao, Clove, Coriander, Cream of Tartar, Cumin, Curry, Dill, Garlic, Plain Gelatin, Horseradish, Marjoram, Mint, Miso, Dry Mustard, Paprika, Red Pepper Flakes, Peppercorn, Peppermint, Rosemary, Saffron, Sage, Sea Salt, Savory, Spearmint, Tamari, Tapioca, Tarragon, Thyme, Turmeric, Wintergreen, Sea Salt

Make sure pre-made condiments are used sparingly and are specifically labeled as Gluten-Free/MSG Free.

BEVERAGES

- Water, Seltzer, Green Tea, Herbal, unlimited
- Red or White Wine, **Gluten-free** Beer: 6 oz

Coffee can be cross-reactive for some folks. Fruit and vegetable juice is best if made at home/fresh but for the sake of controlling blood sugar, avoid fruit juice in general and stick to only eating it. Watch out for flavored waters and juices because these may contain gluten/MSG.

Appendix E:
MSG in Labels-The "Hidden" names for MSG

The following substances contain the highest percentage of factory created free glutamate, with MSG containing 78%:

MSG	Gelatin	Calcium Caseinate
Monosodium Glutamate	Hydrolyzed Vegetable Protein (HVP)	Textured Protein
Monopotassium Glutamate	Hydrolyzed Plant Protein (HPP)	Yeast Extract
Glutamate	Autolyzed Plant Protein	Yeast Food or Nutrient
Glutamic Acid	Sodium Caseinate	Autolyzed Yeast
Vegetable Protein Extract	Senomyx (wheat extract labeled as artificial flavor)	

The following substances contain some factory-created free-glutamate in varying amounts. Please note that some food labels list several of these items, which can add up to a considerable and dangerous amount in one product, or if taken/consumed in several products throughout the day:

Free-glutamate may be in the following:

Malted Barley (flavor)	Natural Flavors, Flavors, Flavoring	Modified food starch
Barley Malt	Reaction Flavors	Rice syrup or brown rice syrup
Natural Chicken, Beef, or Pork, Flavoring "Seasonings" (Most assume this means salt, pepper, or spices and herbs, which sometimes it is)		Malt Extract or Flavoring
Lipolyzed butter Fat	Maltodextrin, dextrose, dextrates	Soy Sauce or Extract
"Low" or "No Fat" Items	Caramel Flavoring (coloring)	Soy Protein
Corn syrup and corn syrup solids, high fructose corn syrup	Citric Acid (when processed from corn)	Soy Protein Isolate or Concentrate
Anything enriched or vitamin enriched	Whey Protein Isolate or Concentrate	Cornstarch fructose(made from corn)
Milk Powder	Bouillon	Flowing Agents
Dry Milk Solids	Carrageenan	Wheat, rice, corn or oat protein
Protein Fortified Milk	Whey Protein or Whey	Stock
Annatto	Broth	Protein Fortified "anything"
Spice	Pectin	Enzyme modified proteins
Gums (guar and vegetable)	Protease	Ultra-pasteurized dairy products
Dough Conditioners	Protease Enzymes	Fermented proteins
Yeast Nutrients	Lecithin	Gluten and gluten flour
Protein powders: whey, soy, oat, rice (as in protein bars,shakes and body building drinks)	Amino Acids (as in Bragg's liquid amino acids and vitamins)	Algae, phytoplankton, sea vegetable, wheat/ barley grass powders

Index

Endnotes

[1] http://www.cdc.gov/pdf/facts_about_obesity_in_the_united_states.pdf

[2] Haag M, Dippenaar NG. Dietary fats, fatty acids and insulin resistance: short review of a multifaceted connection. Med Sci Monit. 2005 Dec;11(12):RA359-67.

[3] Zimmet P; Thomas CR, Genotype, obesity and cardiovascular disease--has technical and social advancement outstripped evolution? J Intern Med - 01-AUG-2003; 254(2): 114-25

[4] H. Pijl, Obesity: evolution of a symptom of affluence Neth J Med, Neth J Med. 2011 Apr;69(4):159-66.

[5] Cordain, Loren, PhD. The Late Role of Grains and Legumes in the Human Diet, and Biomechanical Evidence of their Evolutionary Discordance, United States, 1999. http://www.beyondveg.com/cordain-l/grains-leg/grains-legumes-1a.shtml#celiac.

[6] Wadley, G., Martin, A., The origins of agriculture? A biological perspective and a new hypothesis, Australian Biologist 6: 96 - 105, 1993

[7] Bertrand J., Mars A., Boyle C., et al: Prevalence of autism in a United States population: the Brick Township, New Jersey, investigation. Pediatrics 108. (5): 1155-1161.2001

[8] Steinhausen H.C., Gobel D., Breinlinger M., et al: A community survey of infantile autism. J Am Acad Child Psychiatry 25. (2): 186-189.1986;

[9] Taylor B.: Vaccines and the changing epidemiology of autism. Child Care Health Dev 32. (5): 511-519.2006

[10] Roger, VL et al, AHA Statistical Update: Heart Disease and Stroke Statistics-2011 Update. A Report from the American Heart Association. Circulation, 2011:123: e18-e209.

[11] http://www.cdc.gov/Features/CancerStatistics/

[12] Progress in Autoimmune Diseases Research, Report to Congress, National Institutes of Health, The Autoimmune Diseases Coordinating Committee, March 2005

[13] Hadjivassiliou, M. Sanders, D.S., Grunewald, R.A., Woodroofe, N., Boscolo, S., Aeschilmann, D. Gluten sensitivity: from gut to brain." Lancet Neurol, 2010;9(3):318-330.

[14]Stechschulte SA; Kirsner RS; Federman DG., Vitamin D: bone and beyond, rationale and recommendations for supplementation. - Am J Med - 01-SEP-2009; 122(9): 793-802

[15]Knip M, Akerblom HK. Early nutrition and later diabetes risk. Adv Exp Med Biol. 2005;569:142-50.

[16]Muntoni S, Muntoni S., Gene-nutrient interactions in type 1 diabetes. World Rev Nutr Diet. 2004;93:188-209.

[17]Buchanan HM, Preston SJ, Brooks PM, Buchanan WW. Is diet important in rheumatoid arthritis? Br J Rheumatol. 1991 Apr;30(2):125-34.

[18]Rojahn R., Dietary interventions for rheumatoid arthritis., Am J Nurs. 2011 Mar;111(3):69.

[19]El-Chammas K, Danner E. Gluten-free diet in nonceliac disease. Nutr Clin Pract. 2011 Jun;26(3):294-9.

[20]Tlaskalová-Hogenová H, et al, The role of gut microbiota (commensal bacteria) and the mucosal barrier in the pathogenesis of inflammatory and autoimmune diseases and cancer: contribution of germ-free and gnotobiotic animal models of human diseases. Cell Mol Immunol. 2011 Mar;8(2):110-20.

[21]Fedeles F, Murphy M, Rothe MJ, Grant-Kels JM., Nutrition and bullous skin diseases. Clin Dermatol. 2010 Nov-Dec;28(6):627-43.

[22]Arnson, Y., Amital, H., and Shoenfeld, Y. "Vitamin D and autoimmunity: new aetiological and therapeutic considerations." J of Immunology, 2005, 175: 4119-4126.

[23]Liu Z, Li N, Neu J. Tight junctions, leaky intestines, and pediatric diseases. Acta Paediatr. 2005 Apr;94(4):386-93.

[24]Laukoetter MG, Nava P, Nusrat A., Role of the intestinal barrier in inflammatory bowel disease. World J Gastroenterol. 2008 Jan 21;14(3):401-7.

[25]DeMeo MT, Mutlu EA, Keshavarzian A, Tobin MC. Intestinal permeation and gastrointestinal disease. J Clin Gastroenterol. 2002 Apr;34(4):385-96

[26]Sollid, L.M., Markussen, G. Ek J, Gjerde H., Vartdal, G., Thorsby. Evidence for a primary association of celiac disease to a particular HLA-DQ / heterodimer. J Exp. Med. 1989;169:345-350.

[27] Sollid, L.M., Thorsby, E. HLA susceptibility genes in celiac disease: genetic

mapping and role in pathogenesis. Gastroenterology. 1993;105:910-922.

[28]van der Windt DA, Jellema P, Mulder CJ, et al. Diagnostic testing for celiac disease among patients with abdominal symptoms: a systematic review. JAMA. 2010;303:1738-46

[29]Verdu EF; Armstrong D; Murray JA., Between celiac disease and irritable bowel syndrome: the "no man's land" of gluten sensitivity. Am J Gastroenterol - 01-JUN-2009; 104(6): 1587-94

[30]Barton SH; Murray JA, Celiac disease and autoimmunity in the gut and elsewhere. - Gastroenterol Clin North Am - 01-JUN-2008; 37(2): 411-28, vii

[31]Eswaran S; Tack J; Chey WD., Food: the forgotten factor in the irritable bowel syndrome. Gastroenterol Clin North Am - 01-MAR-2011; 40(1): 141-62

[32]Evans KE, Leeds JS, Sanders DS. Be vigilant for patients with coeliac disease. Practitioner. 2009 Oct;253(1722):19-22, 2

[33]Fasano A, Catassi C. Current approaches to diagnosis and treatment of celiac disease enterology. 2001 Feb;120(3):636-51

[34]Barker JM; Liu E., Celiac disease: pathophysiology, clinical manifestations, and associated autoimmune conditions. Adv Pediatr - 01-JAN-2008; 55: 349-65

[35]Briani C; Samaroo D; Alaedini A., Celiac disease: from gluten to autoimmunity. Autoimmun Rev - 01-SEP-2008; 7(8): 644-50

[36]Ludvigsson, Jonas, F, Leffler, Daniel A, Bai, Julio C, Biagi, Federico, Fasano, Alessio, et. al. The Oslo defintions for coeliac disease and related terms. Gut, 2012, Feb. 16.

[37]Rapin JR, Wiernsperger N. Possible links between intestinal permeablity and food processing: A potential therapeutic niche for glutamine. Clinics (Sao Paulo). 2010 Jun;65(6):635-43.

[38]Uemura, N., et al. Transglutaminase 3 as a prognostic biomarker in esophageal cancer revealed by proteomics. Int. J Cancer, 2009; 124: 2106-2115.

[39]Griffin, M., Casadio, R., Bergamini, C.M. Tranglutaminases: nature's biological glues. Biochem J,2002; Dec 1;(368)377-96.

[40]Kim, S-Y. et al. Tranglutaminases in Disease. Neurochem Intnl, 2002;

40:85-103.

[41]Vermes I., Steur, E.N., Jirikowski, G.F., Haanen, C. Elevated concentration of cerebrospinal fluid tissue transglutaminase in Parkinson's disease indicating apoptosis. Mov Disord, 2004; 19 (10): 1252-4.

[42]Yokoyama, K., Nio, N., Kikuchi, Y. Properties and applications of microbial transglutaminase. Appl Microbiol Biotechnol, 2004; 64 (4): 447-54.

[43]EFSA Panel on Dietetic Products, Nutrition, and Allergies (NDA). Scientific Opinion on Dietary Reference Values for Water. EFSA Journal, ;8(3):1459, 2010

[44]Guarner F, Malagelada JR. "Gut flora in health and disease". Lancet 361 (9356): 512–9, 2003

[45]Pickard KM, Bremner AR, Gordon JN, MacDonald TT. bial-gut interactions in health and disease. Immune responses. Best Pract Res Clin Gastroenterol. 2004 Apr;18(2):271-85.

[46]Lindfors K, Koskinen O, Kaukinen K. An update on the diagnostics of celiac disease. Int Rev Immunol. 2011 Aug;30(4):185-96.

[47]Morita E, Matsuo H, Mihara S, Morimoto K, Savage AW, Tatham AS., Fast omega-gliadin is a major allergen in wheat-dependent exercise-induced anaphylaxis. J Dermatol Sci. 2003 Nov;33(2):99-104.

[48]Sollid, L.M., et al. Antibodies to wheat germ agglutinin in coeliac disease. Clin Exp Immunol, 1986; 63: 95-100.

[49]Kitano, N. et al. Detection of antibodies against wheat germ agglutinin bound glycoproteins on the islet-cell membrane. Diabetic Med, 2009; 5(2): 139-144.

[50]Dalla, Pellegrina, C. et al. Effects of wheat germ agglutinin on human gastrointestinal epithelium: insights from experimental model of immune/ epithelial cell interaction. Toxicol Applied Pharmacol, 2009; 237:146-153.

[51]iPusztai, A. et al. Antinutritive effect of wheat-germ agglutinin and other N-acetylglucosamine-specific lectins. Brit J Nutri, 1993;70:313-321.

[52]Vojdani, A. et al. The immunology of gluten sensitivity beyond the intestinal track. Eur J Inflammation, 2008; 6(2): 47-57.

[53]Vereckei E, Szodoray P, Poor G, Kiss E. tic and immunological processes in the pathomechanism of gluten-sensitive enteropathy and associated

metabolic bone disorders. Autoimmun Rev. 2011 Apr;10(6):336-40.

[54]Farrace, M.G. et al. Presence of anti-tissue transglutaminase antibodies in inflammatory intestinal diseases: an apoptosis-associated event? Cell Death Differentiation, 2001;8:767-70.

[55]Marietta, E.V. et al. Transglutaminase autoantibodies in dermatitis herpetiformis and celiac sprue. J invest Dermatol, 2008; 128:332-335.

[56]Sárdy, M. et al. Epidermal Transglutaminase (TGase 3) is the autoantigen of dermatitis herpetiformis. J Exp Med, 2002;196(6)747-757.

[57]Cascella, N.G., Santora, D., Gregory, P., et al. Increased Prevalence of Transglutaminase 6 Antibodies in Sera From Schizophrenia Patients. Schizophr Bull, 2012, Apr 19.

[58]Jackson, J.R., Eaton, W.W., Casella, N.G., et al. Neurologic and psychiatric manifestations of celiac disease and gluten sensitivity. Psychiatr Q, 2012;83(1)91-102.

[59]Vojdani, A. et al. Immune response to dietary proteins, gliadin and cerebellar peptides in children with autism. Nutri Neuroscience, 2004;7(3):151-161.

[60]Stenberg, R. et al. Autoantibodies to Transglutaminase 6 in children with cerebral palsy. 14th Annual International Coeliac Disease Symposium 2011, Oslo, Norway; Poster Presentation.

[61]Hadjivassiliou, M. et al. Autoantibodies in gluten ataxia recognize a novel neuronal transglutaminase. Ann Neurol, 2008;64(3):332-343.

[62]Aeschlimann, D. et al. Detectional of conformation-specific antibodies to transglutaminase 6 in neurology patients. 14th Annual International Coeliac Disease Symposium 2011, Oslo, Norway; Poster Presentation.

[63]Rosato E; Salsano F., Immunity, autoimmunity and autoimmune diseases in older people. J Biol Regul Homeost Agents - 01-OCT-2008; 22(4): 217-24

[64]Rose NR., Predictors of autoimmune disease: autoantibodies and beyond. Autoimmunity - 01-SEP-2008; 41(6): 419-28

[65]Pastore MR, Bazzigaluppi E, Belloni C, Arcovio C, Bonifacio E, Bosi E, Six months of gluten-free diet do not influence autoantibody titers, but improve insulin secretion in subjects at high risk for type 1 diabetes J Clin Endocrinol Metab. 2003 Jan;88(1):162-5.

[66]Pascolo P, Faleschini E, Tonini G, Ventura A. Type 1 diabetes Acta Diabetol. 2011 Aug 11

[67]Shor DB, Barzilai O, Ram M, Izhaky D, Porat-Katz BS, Chapman J, Blank M, Anaya JM, Shoenfeld Y., Gluten sensitivity in multiple sclerosis: experimental myth or clinical truth? Ann N Y Acad Sci. 2009 Sep;1173:343-9.

[68]Pengiran Tengah CD, Lock RJ, Unsworth DJ, Wills AJ., Multiple sclerosis and occult gluten sensitivity. Neurology. 2004 Jun 22;62(12):2326-7.

[69]Ebert EC, Hagspiel KD., Gastrointestinal and hepatic manifestations of systemic lupus erythematosus J Clin Gastroenterol. 2011 May-Jun;45(5):436-41.

[70]Tian XP, Zhang X., Gastrointestinal involvement in systemic lupus erythematosus, World J Gastroenterol. 2010 Jun 28;16(24):2971-7

[71]Mirza N, Bonilla E, Phillips PE. Celiac disease in a patient with systemic lupus erythematosus Clin Rheumatol. 2007 May;26(5):827-8

[72]Melo FM, Cavalcanti MS, Santos SB, Lopes AK, Oliveira FA., [Association between serum markers for celiac and thyroid autoimmune diseases]. Arq Bras Endocrinol Metabol. 2005 Aug;49(4):542-7.

[73]Lidén M, Kristjánsson G, Valtysdottir S, Venge P, Hällgren R. Self-reported food intolerance and mucosal reactivity after rectal food protein challenge in patients with rheumatoid arthritis Scand J Rheumatol. 2010 Aug;39(4):292-8.

[74]Stenberg P, Roth B, Wollheim FA. Peptidylarginine deiminases and the pathogenesis of rheumatoid arthritis Eur J Intern Med. 2009 Dec;20(8):749-55.

[75]Betterle C, Morlin L. Autoimmune Addison's disease. Endocr Dev. 2011;20:161-72.

[76]Betterle C, Lazzarotto F, Spadaccino AC, Basso D, Plebani M, Pedini B, Chiarelli S, Albergoni M. Celiac disease in North Italian patients with autoimmune Addison's disease. Eur J Endocrinol. 2006 Feb;154(2):275-9.

[77] Stadlmaier E, Spary A, Tillich M, Pilger E. Midaortic syndrome and celiac disease: a case of local vasculitis. Clin Rheumatol. 2005 Jun;24(3):301-4.

[78]Morita E, Matsuo H, Chinuki Y, Takahashi H, Dahlström J, Tanaka A. Food-dependent exercise-induced anaphylaxis -importance of omega-5

gliadin and HMW-glutenin as causative antigens for wheat-dependent exercise-induced anaphylaxis-.Allergol Int. 2009 Dec;58(4):493-8.

[79]Canales P, Mery VP, Larrondo FJ, Bravo FL, Godoy J. Epilepsy and celiac disease Neurologist. 2006 Nov;12(6):318-21.

[80]Boscolo S, Sarich A, Lorenzon A, Passoni M, Rui V, Stebel M, Sblattero D, Marzari R, Hadjivassiliou M, Tongiorgi E. Gluten ataxia: passive transfer in a mouse model. Ann N Y Acad Sci. 2007 Jun;1107:319-28.

[81]Hadjivassiliou M, Rao DG, Wharton SB, Sanders DS, Grünewald RA, Davies-Jones AG.

Sensory ganglionopathy due to gluten sensitivity. Neurology. 2010 Sep 14;75(11):1003-8.

[82]Mittelbronn M, Schittenhelm J, Bakos G, de Vos RA, Wehrmann M, Meyermann R, Bürk K. CD8(+)/perforin/granzyme B(+) effector cells infiltrating cerebellum and inferior olives in gluten ataxia. Neuropathology. 2010 Feb 1;30(1):92-6

[83]Hadjivassiliou M. Immune-mediated acquired ataxias. Handb Clin Neurol. 2012;103:189-99.

[84] Ihara M, Makino F, Sawada H, Mezaki T, Mizutani K, Nakase H, Matsui M, Tomimoto H, Shimohama S. Gluten sensitivity in Japanese patients with adult-onset cerebellar ataxia.,Intern Med. 2006;45(3):135-40.

[85]Ostrowski M, Izdebska M, Grzanka A, Zury A, Grzanka D. [The involvement of transglutaminase 2 in autoimmunological diseases]. Postepy Hig Med Dosw (Online). 2005;59:334-9.

[86]Kárpáti S. Dermatitis herpetiformis. Clin Dermatol. 2012 Jan;30(1):56-9

[87]Antiga E, Caproni M, Pierini I, Bonciani D, Fabbri P. Gluten-free diet in patients with dermatitis herpetiformis: not only a matter of skin. Arch Dermatol. 2011 Aug;147(8):988-9;

[88]Cardones AR, Hall RP 3rd. Pathophysiology of dermatitis herpetiformis: a model for cutaneous manifestations of gastrointestinal inflammation. Dermatol Clin. 2011 Jul;29(3):469-77, x.

[89]Lindqvist U, Rudsander A, Boström A, Nilsson B, Michaëlsson G. IgA antibodies to gliadin and coeliac disease in psoriatic arthritis. Rheumatology (Oxford). 2002 Jan;41(1):31-7.

[90]Hadjivassiliou M, Grünewald RA, Lawden M, Davies-Jones GA, Powell

T, Smith CM.

Headache and CNS white matter abnormalities associated with gluten sensitivity. Neurology. 2001 Feb 13;56(3):385-8.

[91]Roche Herrero MC, Arcas Martínez J, Martínez-Bermejo A, López Martín V, Polanco I, Tendero Gormaz A, Fernández Jaén A.[The prevalence of headache in a population of patients with coeliac disease]. Rev Neurol. 2001 Feb 16-28;32(4):301-9.

[92]Sima H, Hekmatdoost A, Ghaziani T, Alavian SM, Mashayekh A, Zali MR. The prevalence of celiac autoantibodies in hepatitis patients. Iran J Allergy Asthma Immunol. 2010 Sep;9(3):157-62.

[93]Lewis NR, Holmes GK. Risk of morbidity in contemporary celiac disease Expert Rev Gastroenterol Hepatol. 2010 Dec;4(6):767-80

[94]Sestak K, Conroy L, Aye PP, Mehra S, Doxiadis GG, Kaushal D., Improved xenobiotic metabolism and reduced susceptibility to cancer in gluten-sensitive macaques upon introduction of a gluten-free diet, PLoS One. 2011 Apr 12;6(4):e18648.

[95]Anderson LA, McMillan SA, Watson RG, Monaghan P, Gavin AT, Fox C, Murray LJ.

Malignancy and mortality in a population-based cohort of patients with coeliac disease or "gluten sensitivity".World J Gastroenterol. 2007 Jan 7;13(1):146-51.

[96]West J, Logan RF, Smith CJ, Hubbard RB, Card TR.,Malignancy and mortality in people with coeliac disease: population based cohort study. BMJ. 2004 Sep 25;329(7468):716-9. Epub 2004 Jul 21.

[97]Ramos-Remus C, Bahlas S, Vaca-Morales O. Rheumatic features of gastrointestinal tract, hepatic, and pancreatic diseases. Curr Opin Rheumatol. 1997 Jan;9(1):56-61.

[98]Olsen NJ, Prather H, Li QZ, Burns DK. antibody profiles in two patients with non-autoimmune muscle disease implicate a role for gliadin autoreactivity. Neuromuscul Disord. 2010 Mar;20(3):188-91.

[99]Bushara KO. Neurologic presentation of celiac disease Gastroenterology. 2005 Apr;128(4 Suppl 1):S92-7.

[100]Arigo D, Anskis AM, Smyth JM. Psychiatric comorbidities in women with Celiac Disease. Chronic Illn. 2011 Sep 20.

[101]Häuser W, Janke KH, Klump B, Gregor M, Hinz A. Anxiety and depression World J Gastroenterol. 2010 Jun 14;16(22):2780-7.

[102]Juster RP; McEwen BS; Lupien SJ, Allostatic load biomarkers of chronic stress and impact on health and cognition. Neurosci Biobehav Rev - 01-SEP-2010; 35(1): 2-16

[103]Tamashiro KL; Sakai RR; Shively CA; Karatsoreos IN; Reagan LP., Chronic stress, metabolism, and metabolic syndrome. Stress - 01-SEP-2011; 14(5): 468-74

[104]Bailleres. Autoimmunity and Hypothyroidism. Clin Endocrin Metab. 1988 Aug;2(3):591-617.

[105]Larson PR, Ingbar SH: The thyroid gland. In: Wilson JD, Foster DW, ed. Williams' Textbook of Endocrinology, ed 8. Philadelphia: WB Saunders; 1992:367-487.

[106]Karpathios T, Zervoudakis A, Theodoridis C, et al: Mercury vapor poisoning associated with hyperthyroidism in a child. Acta Paediatr Scand 1991; 80:550-552.

[107]Trivalle C, Doucet J, Chassagne P, et al: Differences in the signs and symptoms of hyperthyroidsim in older and younger patients. J Am Geriatr Soc 1996; 44:50-53.

[108]Valentino R, Savastano S, Tommaselli AP, Dorato M, Scarpitta MT, Gigante M, Micillo M, Paparo F, Petrone E, Lombardi G, Troncone R. Markers of potential coeliac disease in patients with Hashimoto's thyroiditis. Eur J Endocrinol. 2002 Apr;146(4):479-83.

[109]Virili C, Bassotti G, Santaguida MG, Iuorio R, Del Duca SC, Mercuri V, Picarelli A, Gargiulo P, Gargano L, Centanni M. Atypical celiac disease as cause of increased need for thyroxine: a systematic study. J Clin Endocrinol Metab. 2012 Mar;97(3):E419-22.

[110]http://www.organic-center.org/reportfiles/5367_Nutrient_Content_SSR_FINAL_V2.pdf

[111]Ahn D, Heo SJ, Park JH, Kim JH, Sohn JH, Park JY, Park J. Clinical relationship between Hashimoto's thyroiditis and papillary thyroid cancer. Acta Oncol. 2011 Nov;50(8):1228-34.

[112]Staii A, Mirocha S, Todorova-Koteva K, Glinberg S, Jaume JC. Hashimoto's thyroiditis is more frequent than expected when diagnosed by cytology which uncovers a pre-clinical state. Thyroid Res. 2010; 3: 11.

[113]Vojdani A. et al. Infections, toxic chemicals and dietary peptide binding to lymphocyte receptors and tissue enzymes are major instigators of autoimmunity in autism. Intl J Immunopathol Pharmacol, 2003; 16(3): 189-199.

[114]Hitoglou M; Ververi A; Antoniadis A; Zafeiriou DI Childhood autism and auditory system abnormalities. Pediatr Neurol - 01-MAY-2010; 42(5): 309-14

[115]Cermak SA; Curtin C; Bandini LG Food selectivity and sensory sensitivity in children with autism spectrum disorders. J Am Diet Assoc - 01-FEB-2010; 110(2): 238-46

[116]Grafodatskaya D; Chung B; Szatmari P; Weksberg R., Autism spectrum disorders and epigenetics. I Am A cad Child Adolesc Psychiatry - 01-AUG-2010; 49(8): 794-809

[117]Nelson P.G., Kuddo T., Song E.Y., et al: Selected neurotrophins, neuropeptides, and cytokines: developmental trajectory and concentrations in neonatal blood of children with autism or Down syndrome. Int J Dev Neurosci 24. (1): 73-80.2006

[118]Pardo C.A., Vargas D.L., Zimmerman A.W.: Immunity, neuroglia and neuroinflammation in autism. Int Rev Psychiatry 17. (6): 485-495.2005

[119]Comi A.M., Zimmerman A.W., Frye V.H., et al: Familial clustering of autoimmune disorders and evaluation of medical risk factors in autism. J Child Neurol 14. (6): 388-394.1999

[120]Martí LF. Effectiveness of nutritional interventions on the functioning of children with ADHD Bol Asoc Med P R. 2010 Oct-Dec;102(4):31-42

[121]Buie T, et al, , Evaluation, diagnosis, and treatment of gastrointestinal disorders in individuals with ASDs: a consensus report. Pediatrics. 2010 Jan;125 Suppl 1:S1-18.

[122]Reichelt KL, Knivsberg AM. The possibility and probability of a gut-to-brain connection in autism. Ann Clin Psychiatry. 2009 Oct-Dec;21(4):205-11.

[123]Elder JH. The gluten-free, casein-free diet in autism: an overview with clinical implications. Nutr Clin Pract. 2008 Dec-2009 Jan;23(6):583-8.

[124]Christison GW, Ivany K., Elimination diets in autism spectrum disorders: any wheat amidst the chaff? J Dev Behav Pediatr. 2006 Apr;27(2 Suppl):S162-71

[125]De Magistris L, Familiari V, Pascotto A, Sapone A, Frolli A, Iardino P, Carteni M, De Rosa M. Francavilla R, Riegler G, Militerni R, Bravaccio C. Alterations of the intestinal barrier in patients with autism spectrum disorders and in their first-degree relatives, J Pediatr Gastroenterol Nutr. Oct;51(4):418-24, 2010.

[126]Weber W; Newmark S., Complementary and alternative medical therapies for attention-deficit/hyperactivity disorder and autism. Pediatr Clin North Am - 01-DEC-2007; 54(6): 983-1006; xii

[127]Knivsberg A.M., Reichelt K.L., Hoien T., et al: A randomised, controlled study of dietary intervention in autistic syndromes. Nutr Neurosci 5. (4): 251-261.2002

[128]Lucarelli S., Frediani T., Zingoni A.M., et al: Food allergy and infantile autism. Panminerva Med 37. (3): 137-141.1995

[129]Washnieski, G.L.,Seaborn, C., Schmidt, C., Nyland, R., Gluten-Free and Casein-Free Diets as a Form of Alternative Treatment for Autism Spectrum Disorders J Am Diet Assoc - September, 2010; 110(9 Suppl 1); A39

[130]Kirby M; Danner E Nutritional deficiencies in children on restricted diets. Pediatr Clin North Am - 01-OCT-2009; 56(5): 1085-103

[131]Mantos,A., Ha, E., Caine-Bish, N., Burzminski,N., Effects of the Gluten-Free/Casein-Free Diet on the Nutritional Status of Children with Autism, J Am Diet Assoc - September, 2011; 111(9 Suppl); A32

[132]http://www.ncbi.nlm.nih.gov/pubmedhealth/PMH0002518/

[133]Nigg JT, Lewis K, Edinger T, Falk M. Meta-analysis of attention-deficit/hyperactivity disorder or attention-deficit/hyperactivity disorder symptoms, restriction diet, and synthetic food color additives. J Am Acad Child Adolesc Psychiatry. 2012 Jan;51(1):86-97.e8.

[134]Breakey J. The role of diet and behaviour in childhood. J Paediatr Child Health. 1997 Jun;33(3):190-4.

[135]Lakhan SE, Vieira KF. Nutritional therapies for mental disorders. Nutr J. 2008 Jan 21;7:2.

[136]Pelsser LM; Frankena K; Toorman J; Savelkoul HF; Dubois AE; Pereira RR; Haagen TA; Rommelse NN; Buitelaar JK., Effects of a restricted elimination diet on the behaviour of children with attention-deficit hyperactivity disorder (INCA study): a randomised controlled trial. Lancet - 5-FEB-2011; 377(9764): 494-503

[137]Pelsser LM; Frankena K; Toorman J; Savelkoul HF; Pereira RR; Buitelaar JK., A randomised controlled trial into the effects of food on ADHD. Eur Child Adolesc Psychiatry - 01-JAN-2009; 18(1): 12-9

[138]Dickerson F, Stallings C, Origoni A, Vaughan C, Khushalani S, Leister F, Yang S, Krivogorsky B, Alaedini A, Yolken R. Markers of gluten sensitivity and celiac disease in recent-onset psychosis and multi-episode schizophrenia. Biol Psychiatry. 2010 Jul 1;68(1):100-4.

[139]Dickerson F, Stallings C, Origoni A, Vaughan C, Khushalani S, Yolken R. Markers of gluten sensitivity in acute mania: A longitudinal study. Psychiatry Res. 2012 Mar 2.(Epub ahead of print).

[140]Rodrigo L, Hernández-Lahoz C, Fuentes D, Alvarez N, López-Vázquez A, González S.

Prevalence of celiac disease in multiple sclerosis BMC Neurol. 2011 Mar 7;11:31.

[141]http://www.ncbi.nlm.nih.gov/pubmedhealth/PMH0002372/ (accessed 10/2011)

[142]Hadjivassiliou M; Sanders DS; Woodroofe N; Williamson C; Grünewald RA., Gluten ataxia. Cerebellum - 01-JAN-2008; 7(3): 494-8.

[143]Alaedini A, Okamoto H, Briani C, Wollenberg K, Shill HA, Bushara KO, Sander HW, Green PH, Hallett M, Latov N. Immune cross-reactivity in celiac disease: anti-gliadin antibodies bind to neuronal synapsin. J Immunol. 2007:6590-5.

[144]Ford RP., The gluten syndrome: a neurological disease. Med Hypotheses - 01-SEP-2009; 73(3): 438-40

[145]Kozanoglu E., Basaran S., Goncu M.K.: Proximal myopathy as an unusual presenting feature of celiac disease. Clin Rheumatol 24. (1): 76-78.2005

[146]Wong M., Scally J., Watson K., et al: Proximal myopathy and bone pain as the presenting features of coeliac disease. Ann Rheum Dis 61. (1): 87-88.2002

[147]Presutti RJ; Cangemi JR; Cassidy HD; Hill DA., Celiac disease. Am Fam Physician - 15-DEC-2007; 76(12): 1795-802

[148]Selby PL, Davies M, Adams JE, et al. Bone loss in celiac disease is related to secondary hyperparathyroidism. J Bone Miner Res 1999;14:652-7.

[149]Kemppainen T, Kroger H, Janatuinen E, et al. Osteoporosis in adult

patients with celiac disease. Bone 1999;24:249-55.

[150]Nuti R, Martini G, Valenti R, et al. Prevalence of undiagnosed coeliac syndrome in osteoporotic women. J Intern Med 2001;250:361-6.

[151]Lindh E, Ljunghall S, Larsson K, et al. Screening for antibodies against gliadin in patients with osteoporosis. J Intern Med 1992;231:403-6.

[152]Becker C Clinical evaluation for osteoporosis. Clin Geriatr Med - 01-MAY-2003; 19(2): 299-320.

[153]Riches PL, McRorie E, Fraser WD, Determann C, van't Hof R, Ralston SH. Osteoporosis associated with neutralizing autoantibodies against osteoprotegerin. N Engl J Med. 2009 Oct 8;361(15):1459-65.

[154]Sbaihi M, Rousseau K, Baloche S, Meunier F, Fouchereau-Peron M, Dufour S. Cortisol mobilizes mineral stores form vertebral skeleton in the European eel: an ancestral origin for glucocorticoid-induced osteoporosis? J Endocrinol. 2009 May;201(2):241-52.

[155]Chiodini I, Scillitani A. Role of corisol hypersecretion in the pathogenesis of osteoporosis. Recent Prog Med. 2008 Jun;99(6):309-13.

[156]Cheng J, Brar PS, Lee AR, Green PH. Body mass index in celiac disease: beneficial effect of a gluten-free diet. J Clin Gastroenterol. 2010 Apr;44(4):267-71.

[157]Ukkola, A.,Mäki, M.,Kurppa, K., Collin, P.,Huhtala, H.,Kekkonen, L., Kaukinen, K., Changes in body mass index on a gluten-free diet in coeliac disease: A nationwide study, European Journal of Internal Medicine (In Press)

[158]Damcott CM; Sack P; Shuldiner AR The genetics of obesity. Endocrinol Metab Clin North Am - 01-DEC-2003; 32(4): 761-86.

[159]Prevalence of overweight and obesity among adults: United States, 1999. National Center for Health Statistics, Center for Disease Control and Prevention Website. Available at: http://www.cdc.gov/nchs/products/pubs/pubd/hestats/obese/obse99.htm (Accessed 1/12)

[160]Camarca, A., Anderson, R.P., Mamone, G., et al. Intestinal T-cell responses to gluten peptides are largely heterogeneous: implications for a peptide-based therapy in Celiac disease. J Immunol, 2009; 182(7):4158-4166.

[161]John P. Reganold, Preston K. Andrews, Jennifer R. Reeve, Lynne

Carpenter-Boggs, Christopher W. Schadt, J. Richard Alldredge, Carolyn F. Ross, Neal M. Davies, and Jizhong Zhou, "Fruit and Soil Quality of Organic and Conventional Strawberry Agroecosystems," Plos ONE, 5, (9), 2010.

[162]http://www.organic-center.org/reportfiles/5367_Nutrient_Content_SSR_FINAL_V2.pdf